D1131638

Freudian Theory and
American Religious Journals
1900-1965

Studies in
American History and Culture, No. 17

Robert Berkhofer, Series Editor
Director of American Culture Programs
and Richard Hudson Research Professor of History
The University of Michigan

Other Titles in This Series

Freudian Theory and American Religious Journals 1900-1965

by
Ann Elizabeth Rosenberg

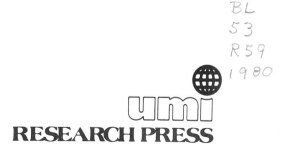

RESEARCH PRESS

Text first published as a
typescript facsimile in 1978

Produced and distributed by
UMI Research Press
an imprint of
University Microfilms International
Ann Arbor, Michigan 48106

Library of Congress Cataloging in Publication Data

Rosenberg, Ann Elizabeth, 1942-
 Freudian theory and American religious journals,
1900-1965.

  (Studies in American history and culture ; no. 17)
  Bibliography: p.
  Includes index.
  1. Psychology, Religious—History. 2. Religious newspapers and periodicals—United States. 3. Freud, Sigmund,
1856-1939. I. Title. II. Series.

BL53.R59 1980   201'.9   80-17544
ISBN 0-8357-1099-8

Contents

Acknowledgments

There are many people without whose help completion of this study would have been impossible. I would like to thank Professor Frederick Kershner for his understanding of the plight of students who are also mothers of young children. I would also like to thank my mother Bertha Schiffer for her endless hours of typing and my husband Norman and my two children, Eric and Joshua, for their cooperation and forbearance. I would like to thank Judah Rackovsky, who worked many long hours on the manuscript. There are many other family members and friends who helped in a variety of ways and to all of them I wish to say thank you.

A.E.R.

Preface

This is a cross-disciplinary study involving the fields of history, religion and psychology. Thus, the study presents special problems with regards to the competency of the writer in all three fields. It is difficult to have equal competency in all fields, and this writer's area of greatest competency is in the field of history both at the undergraduate and graduate levels. The writer also has completed three graduate courses in psychology and two in the field of psychology and religion to provide additional preparation in those areas. This was no hardship since both psychology and religion have been lifelong fields of interest. Thus, while basic preparation has been made in all three areas, the strongest competency is obviously in history, and this study will lean towards a historical approach both by instinct and design.

The writer is quite aware that Freudian psychology is but one of many subareas in psychology, and this is reflected in some of the chapter divisions which follow. If sometimes the term Freudian psychology is used as a shorthand term, this is for literary convenience, and no other reason.

Freud and Religion During the Progressive Era

At the beginning of the twentieth century, when Freud began to record his revolutionary discoveries about the functioning of the human mind, Americans, including all religious groups, were unaware of his work. There was no mention of Freud or of his discoveries in the religious press. Even American physicians working with the mentally ill were unaware of his work. Only a handful of American scholars who had studied and traveled in Europe, where his early writings were available in German, were aware of his pioneering discoveries in the field of psychology.

It was one of those scholars, G. Stanley Hall, who had studied in Europe, and who was an admirer of the German university system and of German science, who introduced Freud's work to the United States.[1] Hall was interested in psychology and was familiar with Freud's writings which were untranslated from the original German. He invited Freud to lecture at the twentieth anniversary celebration of Clark University in 1909.

Freud accepted Hall's invitation and gave a series of lectures at Clark University in German which were reported in the newspapers of the day and which were attended by many leading American psychologists including an ailing William James, the dean of American psychologists, and Jackson Putnam, who founded the American Psychoanalytic Association in 1911 to help disseminate Freud's writings. The Clark lectures were America's first major exposure to Freudian theory. Prior to 1909 Freud's work was virtually unknown in the United States, and psychology in the United States bore almost no resemblance to clinical psychology as we know it today. Unlike anthropology and sociology, in fact, psychology was the youngest of the social sciences to make an impact in America.

Psychology was one of the infant social sciences. The *Journal of Psychology* was founded by G. Stanley Hall in 1887. The new discipline was developed on European, usually German, models.

The leaders of American psychology, such as William James and G. Stanley Hall, studied in Germany, and returned to America impressed with the experimentalism of German science. They established laboratories for testing and measurement in the United States, which were used to study the behavior of animals and children, the process of education, and the workings of the human mind. The primary pattern was that of stimulus and response. All phenomena were to be divided into perceptions, which could be examined and measured. American psychologists observed children at play, and collected data through the use of questionnaires.[2]

Most psychologists were also philosophers. Many were interested in the psychology of religion. The early psychologists were concerned with studying religious experiences in terms of knowledge and of perception. They wanted to obtain scientific verification and explanation of religious experiences, including mystical and conversion experiences. By reducing religion to perceptions subject to scientific verification, early psychologists of religion hoped to establish a scientific proof of the reality of religious phenomena, as distinct from manifestations of mental illness.

William James (1842-1910), an outstanding American philosopher, who was considered the founder of American psychology, formulated the most comprehensive pre-Freudian psychology of religion. James was America's foremost empiricist. He examined and evaluated religious experience in the light of the effects of the experience upon the behavior of the believer.[3]

James rejected other explanations of religious behavior, including those which attributed various manifestations of religious behavior to somatic causes, or to growth and development. He said that religious phenomena such as conversion could only be distinguished from symptoms of mental illness and "diabolical" workings by the test of experience.

James defined religious feelings as normal feelings which were turned towards religious subjects. Man's religion consisted of his feelings, acts, and experiences as he understood himself in relation to whatever he considered to be divine. James included gnostic and naturalistic philosophies in his definition of religion. Religion did not have to be centered around God.

He said that religion was primarily a non-rational experience. It involved the emotions more than the intellect. It was the subconscious and not the conscious mind, the emotions and not the intellect, that were primary in religious experience, including those things which were subliminally perceived.

James judged the health of a soul according to the person's outlook on life. People with healthy souls had either naturally or deliberately optimistic, happy outlooks. Religious convictions gave the possessor feelings of serenity and well being, as well as acting as a prophylactic against disease. The sick soul, on the other hand, was melancholy, and was preoccupied with evil in the world. James was not certain why some people suffered from fewer emotional conflicts, and seemed to live more harmoniously than others. He postulated that those with troubled personalities might have inherited opposing temperaments from different ancestors.

James said that some people were more prone to religious conversion experiences than were others. A person who was subject to dreams and to autosuggestion and was more emotional, was more likely to have a conversion experience. James surveyed the relevant literature on religious conversion. He mentioned J. H. Leuba's discussion of the conversion experience as one that brought a sense of wholeness, peace, and unity to the individual, and which had been preceded by feelings of "unwholeness," sinfulness, and a yearning for peace and unity. There was a feeling of need for a higher helper, and the conversion experience resulted in a sense of being helped.

James said that there were two types of conversion. One was the conscious volitional type, and the other was the self-surrender type, in E. D. Starbuck's terminology, or the conscious voluntary way as opposed to the unconscious involuntary way, according to James.[4] The key element in any conversion experience was the act of yielding, which involved the surrender of the personal will. James said that psychology and religion were in agreement that forces outside the individual brought redemption. The fruits of a conversion experience were often the abolition of a sensual appetite, such as the desire for alcohol.

Conversion experiences were less common in the more traditional branches of Christianity, which placed more reliance on the reception of grace through the sacraments.

James tried to explain the workings of the mind. He said that man had a constant succession of constantly shifting mental fields, which widened and narrowed, and came and departed. At times of religious experience, all of man's senses were flooded with images of the divine. Beyond the field of conscious perceptions lay the memories, suggestions, and dreams which remained on the margin of the conscious self, ready to become conscious when the field of perception shifted to them. The individual was not aware of what lay beyond the conscious self at any particular moment. James said that George A. Coe had found that converts had more active subliminal selves, which were rich in dreams, memories, and suggestions.[5]

According to James, there was general agreement among psychologists of religion that conversion experiences were to be judged by their effect upon the individual. The convert should be a happier, more tranquil person. Physical manifestations of the conversion experience, such as trances or glossolalia, were not proof that the conversion experience was genuine, and not the perceptions of a deranged mind, or the workings of the "diabolical." Few converts experienced serious backsliding, or were subsequently converted to another religion.

James judged saintliness and mysticism by the same criteria with which he judged the convert. Personal characteristics were similar to those of the convert, only more pronounced. James judged saintliness to be good, and not a neurotic manifestation or pattern of religious excesses, because of the behavior of the saints. He noted their peacefulness, happiness, charity, purity, creativity, and lovingness. He excused their excesses as being symptomatic of their age, but noted that they were not infallible, and their utterances, as well as those of the mystics, were to be tested empirically before being accepted.

James suggested that the mystic state was indescribable and known only to the mystic, who attained new insights which transcended the conscious mind or the intellect. He said that the mystic state was transient, and characterized by passivity on the part of the mystic, who surrendered his will to a higher power. The Christian mystic was oriented towards heaven, and was indifferent to worldly things.

James explained his philosophy of religion. He rejected reason as the basis for a philosophy of religion, because reason had to convince all men. James also rejected metaphysical and dogmatic religious philosophies. Neither was the continuance of religious practices through the ages proof of the existence of religion.

He offered the philosophy of pragmatism, because he said that only when thought on a subject had found rest, could belief begin. Thinking was a step in the formation of active habits. He referred to Kant, who had said that conscious thinking had to accompany all subjects. James said that religion had to stand on its own, as part of experience. He said that in a religious person, the conscious mind was continuous with the wider beliefs through which the saving experience came.

James's philosophy was the most comprehensive attempt to understand religion in terms of perceptions and empirical testing. He realized that a large part of the workings of the human mind did not belong to the conscious sphere. He was a believer as Freud offered a new approach to the working of the human mind used to religion. He explained the inner dynamics of the mind in terms of the flow of energy. Freudian psychology was mechanistic and deterministic. The environment was the milieu in which the individual developed and tried to resolve his instinctual conflicts.

Neo-Freudian psychologists placed much more emphasis on the

influence of the environment upon the individual than had Freud, and in that respect they were much more typically American in their outlook. James' empiricism was considered to be uniquely American. Freud and most of the neo-Freudians were not religious. Most were materialistic atheists. They did not recognize the existence of a higher power, nor of divine grace. The basic premises and values of Freudian and neo-Freudian psychologists were quite different.

Some of the later testing of religious attitudes was a continuation of the attempt by early psychologists of religion to measure religious attitudes.[6] However, the overwhelming effort to reconcile psychological and religious knowledge involved clinical and not behavioral or experimental psychology.

E. D. Starbuck tried to differentiate between mystical and non-mystical students. He found little or no difference between them in discrimination, motor skills, sensory responses, simple reaction time, tapping, motor control, or perceptual ability. He did find that mystics were more suggestible, and had inferior skills involving mental effort and ingenuity. But, he warned against drawing too hasty conclusions from his findings.[7]

R. H. Thouless tried to formulate a psychology of religion. He said that there was great difficulty in doing so, because of the lack of scientific knowledge of religion, the lack of trained workers who could collect relevant data, the inaccessibility of laboratory materials, and the lack of adequate methods. He favored studying religion through controlled introspection, studying physio-psychological conditions and statistical analysis and the use of tests and rating scales.[8]

While the psychologists of religion in the United States were attempting to understand religious phenomena in terms of methods and data which could be verified in a laboratory, Sigmund Freud was abandoning his laboratory work in neurology entirely. He rejected late nineteenth and early twentieth century theories of the cause of mental illness, which were that mental illness was caused by lesions in nerves or broken electrical impulses. Neurologists hoped to trace every lesion to its origin in the brain and identify the lesion causing every mental illness. Most people believed that mental illness was an inherited genetic defect.[9] The only way Americans would have learned about Freud in this period was through some articles in journals and periodicals which were of a shallow nature.

Freudian Theory: Implications for Religion

Sigmund Freud,[1] the founder of psychoanalysis, was born in the city of Freiberg, Moravia, in 1856. Raised as a Jew, he was conversant with, if not observant of traditional Jewish customs. He was also exposed to Catholicism.

Freud graduated from the University of Vienna in 1881 with a degree in medicine. In 1885, Freud traveled to Paris to study with the great French neurologist Charcot who used hypnotism in the treatment of mental illness, a departure from accepted medical practice. He married and began to raise a family in 1886.

It was not long before Freud began to diverge from the accepted practice in the treatment of his neurological patients. In 1887 he began to treat his patients by hypnosis. In 1890, Freud tried a psychological approach. He communicated his work first to colleagues, and later to disciples, with almost all of whom he would eventually have somewhat acrimonious partings. They included Josef Breuer, William Fleiss, Alfred Adler, and Carl Jung. Lecturing and publishing, along with his clinical practice, became the dominant activities of Freud's life until he died in London on September 23, 1939.

His first major work, *Studies in Hysteria*, was published in 1890 in collaboration with Josef Breuer, another Viennese neurologist.[2] Breuer ameliorated the symptoms of his hysterical patients, for which there was no demonstrable organic basis, by having them recall, while under hypnosis, incidents from their past, which they otherwise were unable to discuss.

In 1900, Freud wrote the *Interpretation of Dreams*, in which he relied mainly on his own dreams, which he had recorded in the process of his self-analysis. He analyzed each part of his dreams individually and minutely, using the technique of free association, which required the individual to say, or in Freud's case of self-analysis, to record everything which entered his mind, without trying to censor any thought which might seem irrelevant or disreputable.

In 1901, in *The Psychopathology of Everyday Life*, Freud discussed the role of slips of the tongue, errors, omissions, accidents, and humor in everyday life. He said that through these routes, wishes which were otherwise suppressed found expression and interfered with everyday life.

After 1900, Freud explored sexuality, including infantile sexuality. This was his most explosive discovery, to the minds of many people. In 1914, in "On Narcissism", Freud began to consider object relations, by which he meant interpersonal relations, and in 1917, Freud investigated the relationship between mourning and melancholia in a book by that name.

In 1920, Freud revised his libidinal theory of instincts to include two instincts, sex and death. The influence of the carnage of World War I on his theory could be seen in the increased importance given to aggression and the death instinct. The same year, in *Beyond the Pleasure Principle*, Freud considered aggressive impulses to be destructive. In *Group Psychology and the Analysis of the Ego*, in 1921, Freud considered the emotional or libidinal ties which united the church and the army. An important shift in emphasis occurred in the *New Theory of the Mind* in 1923 when he stressed the development of ego psychology as more important than the instinctual theory of character. Ego psychology became the area of greatest development for neo-Freudians.

In 1926, in "The Question of Lay Analysis," Freud addressed himself to the problem of the type of training required for the practice of psychoanalysis. He said that psychoanalysis was a branch of psychology, not of medicine. He felt that medical training for a psychoanalyst was irrelevant.   The analyst had to determine whether the ego was strengthened as a result of treatment and could handle internal and external threats.

Freud wrote several books, including *Totem and Taboo* in 1913, *The Future of an Illusion* in 1927, *Civilization and Its Discontents* in 1930, and *Moses and Monotheism* in 1939, which applied the insights of Freud's psychoanalytic system to the study of society. He discussed aspects of past and present day primitive societies, including biblical society, as well as modern technological society. In general, Freud's forays into social psychology were less successful than his system of psychoanalysis. In some ways, they were easier for the non-specialist to understand than were Freud's works on the psychology of the individual. Freud's studies of society impeded the acceptance of his psychoanalytic insights among religiously oriented readers. His lesser works were used to discredit his major ones.

Although the system called Freudian psychology was basically developed by the early twentieth century, and was modified throughout Freud's psychoanalytic career, certain concepts and methods remained basic to Freudian psychology. One was Freud's division of the human personality into three parts which he called the id, the ego, and the superego. The id consisted of everything with which a person was born including the instincts. It was the source of all energy for the rest of the psychic system, and represented subjective reality. The pleasure seeking id sought the release of tension through reflex action or through primary processes. The ego was the executive of the personality. It mediated between objective reality or the outside world and the demands of the id, and determined how demands were to be satisfied. Lacking a separate existence, it derived its power from the id and sought to satisfy the demands of the id in a socially acceptable manner. The ego was the organized part of the id. The superego functioned as the moral arbiter of the individual. It was the last part of the personality to be formed and reflected the moral standards of the culture as interpreted by the child through the actions of his parents. The conscience of the individual was housed in the superego which included an image of good actions for which he could expect reward and bad actions for which he could be punished. The superego functioned in opposition to the id and to the ego in seeking to deny gratification of instinctual demands, especially those involving sex or aggression, which might conflict with societal demands. The superego tried to mold behavior after an idealized model, while the ego's actions were determined by its perceptions of reality and the id's demands were based upon instinctual needs. Most of time the id, the ego and the superego functioned together as parts of a personality under the leadership of the ego.

The existence of the unconscious was an important discovery. The unconscious was the home of wishes which were repressed and were seeking to be discharged. It was the home of the unbearable idea.

Freud also postulated the existence of instincts which served as the conduits for energy from the body to the id. They supplied the personality with energy. Instincts were psychological representations of physical internal needs such as the need for food. Freud classified the instincts into two groups which he called the life and the death instincts. The life instincts included hunger, thirst, and sex, they were necessary for survival, and their combined energy he called the libido. Since everybody eventually died, Freud postulated the existence of a death instinct, an important derivative of which was aggression, which he considered to be the death instinct turned outward when internally opposed by the life instincts. After viewing the carnage of World War I, Freud placed increased stress on aggression, which he then viewed as rivaling the sex instinct in importance.

Freud said that the personality operated through the distribution and the use of energy by the id, the ego, and the superego. The investment of energy in an object or image by which the id sought to gratify an instinct Freud called an object-choice or an object-cathexis. Identification, another important mechanism, Freud said occurred when the ego acquired energy from the id in order to match a mental image with something in the outside world. When identification occurred, Freud said that the ego had successfully replaced a primary process with a secondary process. The ego also used energy to restrain the id from primary process actions, thereby forming anticathexes, and the dynamics of personality continually involved an interplay of cathexes and anticathexes.

Freud also recognized the existence of anxiety as the response of the ego to overstimulation. He recognized three types of anxiety: real, neurotic and moral. Real anxiety resulted from fear of danger in the real world, and neurotic anxiety was the fear that the instincts would commit some action for which the individual would be punished. Thus, the individual feared that instinctual gratification would lead to punishment. Moral anxiety was generated by the conscience, which feared punishment for actions or for thoughts which violated the internalized moral code. The prototype for all anxiety was the trauma of birth, when the newborn was overwhelmed by stimuli from the external world.

Guilt could be called the innate anxiety felt by an individual before the commission of an act. It was also the feeling of anxiety that could result from an imaginary or a contemplated act. Thus, the relationship of guilt to reality varied. Dynamically, it could be described as the backward flow of the death instinct upon the self. The existence of guilt did not provide a reliable indication of the actual commission of immoral acts. Improved self-understanding, which should result from therapy, in theory reduced guilt feelings and resolved religious problems of scrupulosity.

When the ego could no longer cope with anxiety, it unconsciously utilized irrational defense mechanisms for protection. The principal defense mechanisms were repression, projection, reaction formation, fixation and regression. Repression occurred when a disturbing memory was prevented from becoming conscious, and projection occurred when a source of internal anxiety was attributed to the external world. In reaction formation the person did the opposite of the mandate of the anxiety producing impulse. Fixation occurred when the individual became stuck at one stage of development. Anxiety could cause a fixated person to regress, or go back, to an earlier stage of development.

Freudian psychology was deterministic, postulating that all of man's acts were predetermined by those which preceded them and motivated by instinctual demands. Therefore, just as an individual's life experiences predetermined his passage through his development stages, so an individual's ability to control his actions in conformity with some exterior code of behavior rather than to satisfy instinctual needs, was limited. Viewing man as behaving deterministically was the opposite of viewing him as having free will and responsibility for his action.

Another of Freud's major concepts was that the individual passed through various stages of development within the first five years of life, the critical period for the development of the personality. The first stage he called the oral stage, the second the anal, and the third the phallic. The three stages of development referred to the three erogenous zones producing the most pleasure during each period. Most pleasure originated from the mouth during the oral stage, through sucking and the satisfaction of hunger. The expulsion and retention of feces provided the chief source of pleasure during the anal stage. The chief source of pleasure during the phallic stage was derived from urinating, showing genitalia, and seeing urination. Stimulation was achieved through masturbation.

The Oedipus complex developed during the phallic stage, and continued to affect the personality throughout life. It was the culmination of the child's desire to replace the parent of the same sex as the sexual partner of the parent of the opposite sex, and antagonism towards the parent of the same sex.

Freud considered the Oedipus complex to be one of his most important discoveries, and he elaborated its many ramifications. He said girls and boys experienced the Oedipus complex differently. As infants, children of both sexes loved the mother, who was the chief caretaker, and resented the father as a rival for the mother's affections. The boy feared that the father might castrate him in order to remove him as a rival for the mother's affections; hence, the development of a castration anxiety. The boy then repressed that anxiety by identifying with the father and converted his lustful love of his mother to affection. Freud felt that the superego developed after the resolution of the Oedipus complex.

Girls resolved Oedipus complexes differently. The object of their affections shifted from their mother to their father when they realized that the male possessed a penis. Girls blamed their mother for their castrated condition, thus weakening their bond with her, and in addition, sought to share their father's penis with him. Girls suffered from penis envy instead of castration anxiety, but their resolution of the Oedipus complex was less complete. Although their incestuous desires could never be realized, they were not as fully repressed as were those of boys.

Freud said that from the differences in the resolution of castration anxiety and penis envy, the two aspects of the castration complex, arose the differences between the sexes.

Freud said that at age five, the child passed into a latency period, which coincided with the elementary school years. Sexuality lessened, while other kinds of development occurred. Freud believed that after puberty, mature genital sexuality, combined with other feelings, resulted in marriage to someone who was like the parent of the opposite sex. During the phallic stage new modes of behavior, such as altruism, were possible. While childhood behavior was narcissistic, the adolescent placed more emphasis on socialization. Freud emphasized that human behavior was continuous rather than discontinuous, and modes of behavior from earlier phases of development persisted and were merged with new ones.

While developing analytic technique and utilizing the single case method, Freud also discovered the existence of resistance and transference. In order to undergo successful analysis, a patient had to be able to develop a relationship with his analyst, which enabled him to relive the pathological experiences of his childhood. In doing so, he developed a transference neurosis, which replaced his old neurosis. He could eventually be cured of his transference neurosis. Patients unable to develop a transference neurosis could not be cured. Transference neurosis was tantamount to replay of the patient's Oedipal conflict. Every childhood neurosis was the basis for an adult neurosis and had to be re-experienced as a transference neurosis. Countertransference occurred when the analyst unconsciously transferred his feelings towards another person significant in his life to the patient. Countertransference also hindered analysis.

Freud said that resistance accompanied every step of analysis. Resistance consisted of the defensive forces which opposed analysis and had to be overcome in order for analysis to proceed. Resistance occurred when the patient refused to accept the true nature of his ties to the therapist, and could not accept the real nature of his ties to other people, or his instinctual motivations.

An important belief of Freud's was that all men were psychologically the same, and that the similarities could be demonstrated by psychoanalysis. His theories were based upon classical mythology, and upon scientific works available to him, including Charles Darwin's *On the Origin of Species.*[3] They were not based upon substantial field work by anthropologists, and they did not conform with knowledge subsequently gained from field studies of modern primitive peoples. Therefore, their importance lies in the controversy and antagonism they caused among religious writers, and the resultant great delay in the serious examination of Freud's other theories by them.

In *Totem and Taboo*, in 1913, Freud stated that primitive man lived in "primal hordes" consisting of the father who was the leader, his wives and their children. The father denied access to the females to the younger males, from whom he also required complete obedience. Eventually, Freud believed, the brothers banded together, killed the father, and ate him. The sons felt remorse after the parricide and cannibalistic feast. They decided that this should not recur. They decided not to marry the women, their mothers, and henceforth all marriage partners would be from outside the group, or exogamous. Freud said that the Oedipus complex was a universal phenomenon. The incest taboo was also part of the son's atonement for parricide.

The ritualistic killing and eating of a specially designated animal which was otherwise a forbidden object of consumption was substituted for parricide. This animal became the totemic animal of the clan. Killing of the totemic animal became taboo except under ritually approved circumstances. This feast became an important part of totemic religion. Freud then said that there was a strong relationship between taboo and obsessional neuroses, the label he gave to religion.

In *Totem and Taboo*, Freud offered a psychological explanation of primitive cultures. He claimed that all anthropologists could use his insights into the workings of the human mind to understand other cultures. He saw similarities in the behavior of modern neurotic man and the religious practices of primitive peoples.

Freud thought that society arose to curb man's sexual and aggressive impulses. Freud equated the growth of civilization with the growth of suppression of man's instincts. Civilized man resorted to substitute gratifications including smoking, drug taking, drinking, while others sublimated their feelings through religion and love. In 1927, in *The Future of an Illusion*, Freud called religion an illusion and a mass neurosis. He said that it was a version of wishful thinking, whereby an adult returned to the status of a child in a protected and secure environment. Freud said that through religion, man found authority figures who could help him overcome his feeling of helplessness and the resulting anxiety.

Freud said that religious beliefs represented fulfillment of wishes, originating in the feelings of helplessness of childhood, which were never fully outgrown. Religion could assuage guilt feelings about aggressive impulses. Freud said ceremonial practices gave further comfort. Religion was a neurotic way of handling inevitable human conflicts.

Freud, however, regretted modern man's inability to believe in God. He said that disbelief caused further mental anguish.

Freud considered the life and death of Jesus Christ in *The Future of an Illusion* as a recapitulation of the death of Moses, except that he considered Christianity to be a religion of the son. He said that Judaism was a religion of the father. Christ was the primordial father figure, reborn to be murdered, as had been the leader of the primal horde. Freud explained the trinity as the father, the son and the mob which eventually murdered the father. Since Christ was both the father and the son, his place was less clear than that of Moses, who clearly represented the father figure.

Freud explained anti-Semitism by saying that Jews were taunted with the cry that they had killed God, when in essence what was meant was that they had killed their father. The accusation of parricide was correct, according to Freud's psychoanalytic interpretation of the Mosaic and the Christ stories. Freud felt that the biblical injunction to love thy neighbor as thyself was psychologically impossible. He believed that self-centeredness was inevitable, and the legitimacy of the aggressive instinct had to be recognized.

In 1930, in *Civilization and its Discontents,* Freud discussed the instinctual nature of aggression, which he felt was the most powerful obstacle to culture. Of all instinctual privations, Freud felt that the deprivation of the aggressive instinct was the most difficult. He felt that, although cultures tried to mitigate the suffering which occurred because of renunciation of aggression, some suffering was inevitable. Civilizations tried to check aggressiveness by internalizing, or introjection. The renunciation of aggression was always accompanied by guilt. Freud said that modern man internalized aggression through education, and the internalization of aggression resulted in heightened guilt as the individual sought to mediate between his instinctual demands and the demands of society. He said that the prevailing sexual morality of his day resulted in nervous illness.

In *Moses and Monotheism,* in 1939, Freud explained the story of Moses according to psychoanalytic understandings. He said that Moses was an Egyptian who worked for the Egyptian Pharoah Ikhnaton. Ikhnaton tried to impose monotheism on Egypt. After his death, his religious revolution was undone. According to Freud, Moses, the Egyptian, then turned to the Semitic peoples in Egypt. They accepted Moses as their leader, and they also accepted the puritanical form of monotheism he preached. After a while, the Semites tired of the new religion. They murdered Moses, and adopted the Midianite rite of worship of Jahve. However, the religion of Moses eventually triumphed.

Jahve became the omnipotent, loving and just father figure. The God of Moses and the ideals of Moses triumphed after his death. The Semites felt remorse after Moses' murder. They gradually accepted the puritanical worship of the monotheistic God. Freud felt that Christ was a recapitulation of Moses, and Christ's death only a replay of Moses' martyrdom.

Although Freud elaborated a system for understanding and analyzing the workings of the human mind which he constantly revised, many areas were not fully explored, and possibly a complete exploration of the human mind was impossible in one lifetime. Post-Freudians examined Freud's work, making modifications and additions. Some of the areas which have received greater attention by the neo-Freudians are the oral stage of sexuality, along with the mother-child relationship, which was considered to be critical during this stage. All the libidinal stages have been explained more fully. Object relations or interpersonal relations have been closely scrutinized. There has been more study of all types of neuroses. There has been increased interest in psychosomatic medicine and the relationship of mental illness to society. In the post–World War II era, psychoanalysis has become better integrated into general psychology.

Neo-Freudian Theory:
Implications for Religion

Freud's theories were revised and developed by his colleagues, Alfred Adler and Carl Gustav Jung, and his first generation European disciples, Otto Rank, Wilhelm Reich, Melanie Klein, and Anna Freud, and later by second generation neo-Freudians such as Karen Horney, Erich Fromm and Harry Stack Sullivan, an American. The last three worked extensively in the United States. The theories of the neo-Freudians were often more widely known and accepted than Freud's theories because the neo-Freudians often worked hard at popularizing their ideas, and they were often more concerned with contemporary problems such as anxiety, loneliness and alienation.

Alfred Adler (1870-1937) was the first of Freud's disciples to reject certain elements of Freud's work and offer his own modification of analytic psychology.[1] He developed Individual Psychology, which he considered to be holistic and humanistic, as opposed to Freudian psychology, which was mechanistic, and spoke of drives in conflict with one another. Stressing man's creative and cognitive abilities, his free will and his freedom of choice, he said that man was indivisible and unique. All functional mental disorders were mistaken ways of living, and could be cured by showing a patient his undesirable goals and life applications, and how he could improve them. Individual Psychology was pragmatic and optimistic. It fit the American dream and outlook much more closely than did the mechanistic, deeply introspective, deterministic, conflict-filled and sex-ridden Freudian psychology.

The Adlerian approach stressed the conscious mind or ego psychology. People were seen as organisms striving towards superiority and conquest in order to overcome feelings of inferiority which originated in the dependence of childhood. Inferiority could be resolved in three possible ways. The individual could successfully compensate for his feelings of inferiority through work and sex; he could compensate for his feelings of inferiority, but then his strivings for superiority would become too apparent and offensive to other people. Or he could retreat into illness in order to gain power over others.

Believing that the will to power was the strongest instinct, Adler divided people into four categories based upon social interest and degree of activity. These were high social interest–high activity, which he called the ideally normal; low social interest–high activity, which resulted in a tyrannical or delinquent personality; low social interest–low activity, which was characteristic of someone who, wanting to get things from others, leaned upon others and avoided doing things. Some neurotics and psychotics fitted into this category. The final type displayed high social interest and low activity. Significantly, these categories were much easier for laymen to understand than was Freudian terminology.

Without attempting to explain the causation of every symptom, he offered a theory of psychopathology in which he argued that everyone lived in a world of his own construction in accordance with his perceptions. More serious errors in perceptions might be called symptoms which were creations used to avoid facing life's problems and to free the person from responsibility. Every symptom said something about the organism as a unified whole. Every person was partly right, in that the symptom explained something that had happened to him, but only incompletely. Other people dealt with the same experiences in another way. The neurotic had to understand that he could react to his experience in a non-neurotic way, by seeing the difference between his private perceptions and the common sense perceptions of others in the world around him. Anxiety and phobias prevented the person from doing things which might lead to defeat, Adler cautioned. However, anxiety made it harder for a person to fulfull his life tasks; once a pattern was acquired it was usually maintained. Anxiety also drained a person's energy, leaving him little to expend on others, and, therefore, lowering him on the scale of social action.

Not believing that there were many different mental illnesses, he felt that all mental disorders were the outcome of mistaken ways of living by discouraged people with strong feelings of inferiority, who developed rigid methods for attaining superiority. Psychoses such as schizophrenia or manic depression were not considered as being different from neuroses, only more extreme. He said that psychoses and neuroses shared the same compulsive symptoms, and were variants on extreme superiority complexes. The schizophrenic had abysmally low self-esteem, which he balanced by extravagant goals of superiority, accompanied by a loss of all interest in others, as well as in his own reasoning and understanding. Not interested in dream analysis and feeling that dreams related only to current life problems, Adler examined a patient's attitudes and behavior and their consequences. Both were examined on a more superficial level than by Freud.

The schizophrenic exhibited the low social interests mentioned in

Adler's prototypes. Hallucinations, which sometimes occurred in psychotic stages, were attempts to have something or make something happen without taking any responsibility for the actions. They were also connected to the feelings of superiority. Through hallucinations, subjective impulses could appear to become reality. Perversions resulted from the distance between men and women, and the resulting anxiety.

Viewing suicide and depression as attempts to force one's will upon others by anticipating one's ruin, without taking responsibility for one's actions, he considered adolescent suicide as an act of revenge, and all neuroses as devices for torturing others. The manic state, which often accompanied feelings of depression, was an attempt at superiority to cover feelings of inferiority. Manics and depressives lacked self-confidence and appreciation of others, whom they seemed to exploit.

Neuroses occurred when the drive for superiority was diverted into other channels consonant with the personality structure, whereby the person could avoid a situation which could cause a blow to his prestige.

In the process of therapy, the patient was encouraged to reconstruct the goals and assumptions of his world in terms of greater social usefulness and in closer approximation to the perceptions of others. The patient was shown the goals of personal superiority which resulted from his feelings of inferiority. The therapist first attempted to establish a good relationship with the patient. Next, he gathered information from the patient about his past in order to better understand him, and to obtain material to enable the therapist to conceptualize the lifestyle of the patient. The therapist then tried to interpret the data, and lastly tried to communicate his interpretations to the patient, and enable the patient to change his lifestyle. Adler felt that the patient could consciously and meaningfully cooperate as an equal with his therapist, and could change his behavior without really understanding the factors motivating the change. In this area, Adlerian therapy, which he called individual therapy, agreed with behaviorism.

Adlerian therapy was pragmatic and eclectic, employing a variety of methods, including drug therapy and electric shock therapy, to break through into the patient's private world, and bring the patient into increased contact with other people.

The therapist would confront the patient with the patient's role in his life situation, and make suggestions as to how the patient could improve his behavior, or try to provoke the patient into action by saying that the patient should continue as he was, bearing in mind the consequences of his past actions.

Emphasizing the environment and the effort that a patient made in any direction, he named his psychology Individual Psychology, because of his emphasis on the individual, including his unique goals, purposes, and intentions. Adler felt that the individual possessed almost unlimited creativity with which he fashioned his world, and that a man had to understand his own goals, and the fact that he created them, in order to successfully control his own behavior.

Adler was a tireless lecturer, and a prolific writer of popularized optimistic psychoanalytic literature during the last two decades of his life. The early reception of his work and writings was far more favorable than that of Freud. Today, however, there are few formal Adlerians, although his influence can be seen in the work of some psychologists, including Rollo May, Victor Frankel, O. Hobart Mowrer, Karen Horney, and Ian Suttie.

Carl Gustav Jung (1875-1961) was a Protestant Swiss doctor and psychoanalyst.[2] The only Christian in Freud's original circle of disciples, he combined his extensive knowledge of philosophy, mythology, and anthropology to create a psychology which differed from Freudian psychology in many areas.

Jung introduced a number of new concepts, including the concepts of the ego, the persona, and the shadow. In a mature person the ego acted as mediator between the internal and external worlds. The persona acted as a mask, indicating the roles people played in the outside world. The shadow was the aspect of the ego which dealt with the inner world. The shadow might be compensatory, having characteristics which the person lacked. It was at the doorway to the unconscious, and might reveal an archetypical aspect of the person.

In dividing the unconscious into the personal and the collective unconscious, he said that the personal unconscious contained everything forgotten, repressed, subliminally perceived, thought or felt. The collective unconscious was shared by all humanity. It contained mythological associations, motifs, and images which were universal and timeless. The conscious mind balanced the unconscious; it contained what was lacking in the unconscious mind. In his later years, he revised his theory to state that a unity existed between the conscious and the unconscious mind.

Every Jungian complex had a shell and a core. The shell represented the surface, and the core the archetypical content. The shell of a complex consisted of a pattern of reactions grouped around a central personal emotion. The core of a complex was archetypical, containing a theme found in mythology. An archetypical idea resembled a fantasy or an idea containing a specific behavior pattern more than a hallucination.

Jung thought that man progressed by improving the ethical and spiritual content of archetypical behavior.

He introduced the concepts of anima and animus, which were inner attitudes represented in the unconscious by the image of a definite person, who had qualities lacking in the conscious personality. The anima was feminine, and was to be found in males, while the animus was male and was to be found in females.

The self, which he described as being in contrast to the ego mediator, contained the whole range of psychic activity. Individual differences arose as people tried to reconcile the demands of society with individual needs. People were divided into extroverted and introverted types. The energies of the introvert flowed back upon himself, while those of the extrovert flowed towards the world.

Describing intuition and thinking as sensations, he called intuition perceptions via the unconscious which were directed inward or outward, depending upon whether the person was an introvert or an extrovert. Thinking was divided into thinking about objective data and about subjective data. Objective data was extroverted while subjective data was introverted. A balance existed between the two types of thinking. Extroverted feelings and values were traditional, and generally represented the traditional social standards of the society.

Placing limited importance on sexuality, and denying that all pleasure was really sexual pleasure, Jung called the libido a nonsexual life force having three stages. The first stage lasted from three to five years, during which sexual concerns centered around nutrition and growth. The second stage was a period of prepubic latency which was followed by the third and lasting period of mature sexuality. Jung de-emphasized the Oedipus and castration complexes. He said that the Oedipus complex was founded upon a primitive love for the food-producing mother. This love took on a sexual tinge only during the prepubertal phase. He characterized the castration complex as a symbolic renunciation of infantile wishes, having little or nothing to do with actual castration.

Interpreting dreams as attempts at compensation rather than as wish fulfillment, his view of man was more compensatory and balanced rather than regressive and conflict-oriented. Delving into the past itself seemed regressive.

More interested in older people than was Freud, he claimed that all persons over thirty-five years of age showed signs of anxiety over the finitude of life, while they continued to grow and to develop as they wrestled with problems of meaning, and developed new syntheses which were appropriate to old age. He thought that the absence of religion was the chief cause of psychoses in people over thirty years of age.

Saying that any belief, such as belief in God, which had great emotional significance for a person, must in some sense be true, he offered a subjective definition of truth, which contrasted with objective truth as defined by scientists.

The *Dasein* and existentialist schools of psychology of religion were influenced by Jung. Religious people shared Jung's interest in the problems of mortality, and the crisis engendered by them.

His most generally accepted work was the development of the word association test used to trace the development of complexes, especially in psychotic patients and in schizophrenics in particular. Freud had confined his work almost entirely to neurotics. Jung was also able to produce descriptions of temperaments such as introvert and extrovert.

Jungian therapy was a combination of Freudian and Adlerian methods. In the first stage, confession, the therapist listened to the life history of the patient, and determined the method of treatment. In the second stage, the information provided by the patient was interpreted, putting special emphasis on any transference which had occurred. This emphasis on the importance of transference showed Freudian influence. In the third stage, the patient was educated as to how he could better meet the demands of society. This stage showed Adler's influence. In the last stage, the person tried to transform himself, or let himself grow into a new and healthier individual. This was called individualization. Jung favored shorter periods of therapy than did Freud, thereby allowing the patients time to try to manage their own lives, and lessening the danger of a patient's becoming too dependent upon the therapist.

Many others of the original Vienna Psychoanalytic Society differed with Freud in some aspect of theory or practice. Freud's disciples often made significant discoveries which were utilized by third generation practitioners to further improve the art of psychoanalysis.

Otto Rank (1884-1939) broke with Freud because he believed that the birth trauma, not the Oedipus complex, was the most anxiety provoking experience.[3] He was the first psychoanalyst who was not a medical doctor, and he too tried to shorten the time necessary for therapy by limiting analysis to current problems without delving into the patient's past. This was ultimately not successful. Rank was a Marxist, and he felt that Oedipal conflicts were tied to western capitalist society, and would end with the abolition of class conflicts.

He stressed the importance of the mother-child relationship in the development of the child. The mother nurtured and protected the child, and the child developed a dependency on her which was entirely natural. There were other instincts as important as the sex instinct, such as primal anxiety, which included fear of life, death, fear of losing one's individuality, and of losing one's existing relationships by realizing one's creative potential. Primal anxiety could be resolved in two ways that were not neurotic, or it could be resolved neurotically. An individual could accept the standards of the group, and be rewarded with many relationships while surrendering his creative potential. Or, he could act independently and creatively, ignoring group standards. The neurotic, however, could neither act creatively nor accept group standards.

Rank's greatest contributions were considered to be his emphasis on the mother-child relationship, which influenced anthropologists and psychologists, and his emphasis upon cultural factors. Karen Horney and Clara Thompson were two third-generation psychoanalysts who were influenced by Rank.

Melanie Klein (1882-1960) accepted most of Freudian theory, and is best known for her work with young children and her theory of object splitting.[4] Employing play therapy to reach a silent child, she developed pure transference analysis by discarding all forms of reassurance and all attempts to instruct the patient about the proper way of life, and limiting herself to analyzing the picture of the analyst as it occurred and changed in the patient's mind.

Although willing to begin the treatment of a child at the age of two years, she did not involve the parents in the analysis of their child, because they could not give reports of the child's behavior which were not distorted by their own unconscious conflicts. In general, Klein did not attach much importance to the child's life experiences; instead, she analyzed the child's fantasies.

In describing the acts of object splitting and projection with regard to the mother's breasts, she said that the child perceived the breast as good and loving when the breast provided satisfaction and food. The child hated the breast when it failed to provide satisfaction and projected that hate onto the breast, thinking that the breast hated him. She believed that the Oedipus complex began much earlier in life than Freud had thought, and said that infants perceive the parents as unified. The child's earliest depressive stage was caused by the fear that the child had killed the good parents because of his lust and greed. The infant's superego was modeled after the chastising parent. Freud had dated the development of the superego from the dissolution of the Oedipus complex, which Klein placed in early childhood.

According to Kleinian theory, the roots of schizophrenia were in childhood.   The person who could not tolerate the depressed state of mourning regressed to the schizophrenic state.   Psychoanalysis, according to Klein, had to extend back into a patient's infancy in order to be complete.   Analysis had to include the patient's earliest feelings of anxiety and aggression.

Anna Freud (b. 1895) was Sigmund Freud's youngest child; she devoted her life to extending her father's work in the areas of ego and child psychology.[5]

During World War II, she worked in a nursery with children who were separated from their parents. Finding that the separation from the mother caused the child to develop inhibitions and to regress to an earlier state of development, she said that the environment affected the instinctual life of children, acting through the child's ego. Once a child established a stable relationship with another woman, who acted as a surrogate mother, the symptoms disappeared, and the child continued to progress.   Therefore, good object relations were necessary for normal human development and the control of aggressive impulses.   She concluded that object relations with the mother preceded the Oedipal conflict, and were more important to the child's development than the Oedipal complex.

Theorizing that psychoanalysis was more than analysis of the id through free association and dream analysis, she said that the analysis of defense   mechanisms   such   as   reaction   formation,   sublimation, rationalization, displacement, and projection was necessary to understand the transformations which instinctual drives had undergone, and the restrictions they placed on the ego. Most of her observations concerned children, but she felt that they were equally operative in adult behavior.

She believed that a child's superego began as generalized anxiety about the environment, and was stricter than the superego of an adult, because children introjected the superegos, but not the more tolerant conscious attitudes, of the parents.

Using the methods of orthodox Freudian analysis, she only analyzed children whose speech was adequately developed to enable them to cooperate verbally in their analysis. She introduced flexibility into the analytic situation by allowing children to tell stories and play games, while gradually interpreting the stories and the games for the children, and being especially careful to protect the immature ego of the child, which was still primarily concerned with controlling primitive instincts.

She adapted the techniques of psychoanalysis to the strengths and needs of children, while seeking to form an educative relationship which would enable them to accept a therapist's interpretations. She pioneered in the use of play therapy with children, theorizing that children could not free associate to form true transference neuroses, because they were still too tied to their parent, and were reacting to the present situation, not just to past experience. She tried to work with the parents, upon whom she relied to bring the child regularly, to report on the child's progress and behavior and to enable the analyst to understand how the child's personality developed at home. Sometimes changes in a child's environment were sufficient to eliminate some of the child's symptons.

Melanie Klein and Anna Freud did pioneering work with children. Although they sometimes differed in the techniques they employed, and in their theoretical formulations, they presented a view of the personality of children which differed greatly from the traditional Judeo-Christian view. Both Klein and A. Freud pictured the psyche of the child fighting to control aggressive and sexual impulses at very young ages. The traditional religious views of children emphasized their innocence and idyllic quality, often picturing them as little angels or lambs.

W. R. D. Fairbairn of Edinburgh (b. 1889) continued the development of ego psychology in the area of object relations.[6] His work has had a profound influence on present day psychoanalytic practice. Giving an entirely psychoanalytic explanation of the workings of the mind, and abandoning the mechanistic formulations of Freud's libidinal drives and psychological structures, he said that everyone was born psychologically unblemished and whole, however, the ego lost its natural unity as the result of early bad object relationships. The prime libidinal drive was the ego's search for good object relations, which made ego strength possible. Characterizing aggression as a reaction to the thwarting of the libidinal drive, his definition was similar to Freud's later definition of anxiety as a defense against a threat to the ego.

The sexual development of the individual was divided into three phases: an immature dependence in infancy, a transitional phase, and a mature dependence on an adult level. Neuroses and psychoses were explained as attempts of the ego to defend itself against internal threats of an external origin.

Klein had studied object splitting in object relations, and Fairbairn extended Klein's theory of object splitting to ego splitting, while emphasizing the importance of object relations in the mother-child relationship.

The ego, which was the principle psychic structure, was divided into three parts. The first part, the central ego or the "I," was similar to the Freudian ego. However, it was a dynamic structure, which was not dependent upon energy or impulses from the id. The other egos were derived from the primary ego. The libidinal ego roughly corresponded to the Freudian id and was more infantile than the primary ego. The third ego, which he characterized as aggressive and persecutory, was the internal saboteur. The ego was continually striving to reach objects where it could gain support, reach its full potential, and attain security. The schizoid ego, in contrast, was weak and helpless.

The value of psychotherapy, according to Fairbairn, was that psychotherapy provided an opportunity for the ego to mature through the development of good relationships. During the analytic process, the analyst had to survive the patient's projecting bad internal objects onto him.

Harry Stack Sullivan (1892-1948), an American psychologist,[7] was best known for his work with schizophrenics and adolescents. He divided personality development into six epochs. The first was infancy, during which the infant realized his own capacity. Parents imprinted their personalities onto their children during infancy, when child and mother were particularly empathetic. A unique affective state existed at this time between mother and child. In the second phase, a child acquired language and received cultural indoctrination. Clashes between the interest of children and of parents now appeared. During the latency or juvenile phases, belonging to and cooperating with a peer group became very important to the child. The fifth stage was pre-adolescence, during which the early stages of puberty occurred. The child changed from being egocentric to becoming fully social as friendships became as important as one's self. The final stage was adolescence, which he divided into early, middle, and late phases. The outcome of adolescence was the establishment of periods of intimacy.

Seeing man as being in constant pursuit of the satisfaction of biological needs, which must be achieved in a culturally approved manner, he attributed feelings of being bad, of discomfort, and of in-security to the failure to satisfy needs and to attain power in inter-personal relations.

The individual's attitude towards others were determined by his attitude toward himself. His self-awareness arose from anxiety. The individual sought freedom from anxiety and security in all circumstances, by dealing with all threats towards the self by anger and sublimation. When the self was hateful, all friendly experiences were misinterpreted.

He agreed with Freud that complex motivational systems existed in disassociation from the self, and might find expression in dreams, errors, fantasies and interpersonal relations. The areas of the self to which we were selectively inattentive, he called the selective unconscious. The true unconscious was beyond the selective unconscious.

Interaction with others required the achievement of satisfaction. Biological needs were zonal and caused tension in the individual, while satisfaction could only be achieved in cooperation with others. The child organized himself into a "good me" and a "bad me." The "bad me" was formed as the result of all experiences which elicited an anxious response in his parents, and hence in himself. The "good me" was formed as the result of impulses which resulted in euphoria from satisfactions. Extreme anxiety-producing experiences, which could not be dealt with by selective inattention, were disassociated from the self. They could not be consciously recalled, but might reappear during adolescence or other critical periods. He said that the "good me" and the "bad me" were integrated into the "me" after the child acquired language. Situations causing catastrophic anxiety were dealt with as "not me." The feelings of "not me" were experienced in the face of strong parental anxiety, at adolescence, in nightmares, or as feelings of awe, dread or loathing.

Believing that the therapist was an active participant in the psychoanalytic process, he began by taking an extensive history of the patient's past life, and assembling all information about the patient and his goals. He helped the patient discover the disassociated "bad me" and reintegrate it into the personality. The goal of psychotherapy would be to enable the reintegrated individual to develop mature satisfying object relations.

Wilhelm Reich (1897-1957) linked bourgeois sexual morality to the rise of fascism in Europe.[8] He said that the authoritarian structure of the bourgeois family led to repression of sexual desires in the child, and to the Oedipus complex. All neurotics suffered from a disturbance of the genital function, while sexual taboos led to a further and more general repression of desires. A pattern of submission and repression developed within the individual as he became accustomed to submission to the authoritarian state. Reich said that submission was unhealthy, because it led to mental illness and to political totalitarianism. These social theories influenced Karen Horney and Erich Fromm.

Reich's pioneering work in analytic theory was in the field of character disorders, which he described as the adjustments the ego made to the instincts and to the external world. He said that character disorders were a specific form of neurosis.

Karen Horney (1885-1952), a German psychoanalyst who migrated to the United States, was interested in the integrated whole of the human being, which could only be developed in a social milieu.[9] She said that neuroses were culture bound forms of development generated by a specific set of incidents under specific cultural, not biological, conditions. All neuroses were caused by fears, and were attempts to find compromise solutions for conflicting tendencies originating in childhood.

Denying that there was any universally normal behavior, because anthropological studies had shown that normal behavior in different cultures varied widely, she said that behavior which was normal in one culture might be considered neurotic in another. All neurotics, however, showed rigidity in their reactions, and discrepancies between their potentialities and their accomplishments. A particular form of behavior or trait would be considered neurotic for an individual if it was used to solve an intrapsychic conflict, even though it might be considered normal in other cultures.

An individual had to love and respect himself for what he actually was, in order to love and respect others. Conflicts were rooted in modern industrial culture, although the energy put into the conflicts came from the basic anxiety of childhood, which in turn originated in feelings of isolation and helplessness in a hostile menacing world. A child's ability to handle this basic anxiety depended upon the treatment received from the parents. A parent whose behavior alternated between idealization, indulgence and unrealistic expectations on the one hand and hostility and disparagement on the other hand was particularly destructive to the child's ability to deal with anxiety. The stronger the feelings of anxiety grew, the more rigid behavior patterns became, which in turn resulted in detachment and withdrawal, in addition to or combined with neurotic demands for affection and power. The unresolved neurotic conflicts caused self-alienation, a split between the actual and the idealized self.

Horney differed from Adler in that she felt that not all strivings for power were neurotic. Some represented superior interests or abilities on the part of the individual. A neurotic individual felt that he was entitled to have his neurotic demands satisfied with no effort on his part. He hated himself, because his actual self fell short of the demands his idealized self made upon the actual self. His hate led to further alienation.

Viewing self-alienation as life's crucial problem, she saw two types of alienation. Alienation from the actual self appeared symptomatically, as hysteria and depersonalization. The second type of alienation was alienation from the real self, resulting in the impairment of spontaneous feelings, with less energy available for self-realization and difficulty in making choices and in integrating needs.

Religious leaders were very interested in Horney's views on the effects of alienation, because they felt that religion provided the vehicle through which feelings of anxiety could be allayed, and problems of alienation cured.

Erich Fromm (1900-1980), a European-trained analyst who continued his career in the United States, was influenced by Freud, Rank and Marx, and corresponded with Horney and Sullivan.[10] Primarily interested in the relationship between the individual and the society, and especially in the individual's ability to transcend that society, he was part of a trend in American social psychology which regarded the individual as an offshoot of the society.

Freud had said that the fundamental problem of neurosis arose from the libido seeking satisfaction and often coming into conflict with society's demands. Thus, the fundamental problem of neurosis arose from the relationship of the individual to his society, which was continually changing, and the individual's irrational strivings to fulfill his needs. Societies, he said, have not only suppressed drives but have created what was called human nature.

Fromm turned to history for an explanation of modern neuroses. He believed that society was molded by the continuous interaction between man and society. The main problem of psychology was to determine how the individual related to the society, to the world, and to himself. Believing that personality changes had occurred as society changed, he said that man first had to relate to nature, then to a corporate social order. In the Middle Ages, all people belonged to the social order, in which they occupied a fixed and easily discernible place, and whose framework was devotion to the loving mother church. The problem with the modern social order was that it lacked a definite framework. Since there was no universal framework or orientation and devotion, the individual was unable to impose any rational order upon himself, in order to explain his relationship to himself, to his fellow man, or to the world in general. Modern man was, therefore, beset by intolerable feelings of helplessness and loneliness.

The psychic mechanism by which man tried to escape from this loneliness resembled Horney's neurotic traits. There were three ways of escaping from modern helplessness and isolation: moral masochism and sadism, destructivism, automation and conformity. Moral masochism corresponded to the neurotic need for affection, and was accompanied by feelings of inferiority and inadequacy, along with the need to be dependent upon others in a weak and helpless manner. Often disguised as love and devotion, it really represented a neurotic compulsion and not real affection or love. Sadism was the reverse of masochism and almost always accompanied it. Similar to Horney's neurotic striving for power, it involved the wish to make others dependent upon oneself, to exploit others, or make them suffer mentally or physically. A destructive and authoritarian person was not completely different from a masochist. He tried to escape from unbearable feelings of powerlessness and isolation, contrasting with the power and unity of the world around him, by trying to destroy the surrounding world. Automation and conformity, the last way of dealing with the modern world, resembled Horney's submissiveness. None of these patterns could be described as entirely productive or destructive; all were mixtures.

All societies formed certain character types. One type, the receptive character, believed that all good things, such as knowledge, pleasure and love, came from outside the individual, and should be passively accepted. The receptive character had a great fondness for food and for drink and related to others as a moral masochist. Although he needed to be loved, he could not love, and he needed a magical helper which could be God. He was identical to Freud's oral type.

The exploitative character satisfied all demands in an aggressive manner, by force and cunning, and preferred stealing to producing. This individual had a neurotic need for power, and could be characterized as an oral, aggressive character, who related to others sadistically. The exploitative type believed that all good came from outside of himself, as did the receptive character.

The hoarding character was punctual, pedantic, and sought to insulate himself from the world. Fromm's hoarding character corresponded to Horney's type showing neurotic withdrawal and to Freud's anal erotic type. His security was based upon what he saved or possessed, not upon what he loved. Fromm felt that the hoarding character was typical of the bourgeois economy of the eighteenth and nineteenth centuries.

The family was the socializing agent. A child needed warmth and encouragement from the parents, whose personalities, rather than the method of child rearing, determined the mental health of the child. The process of individuation should accompany growth at a normal rate. If there was a lag in individuation and in growth, loneliness and anxiety developed, and the child tried unsuccessfully to recapture primary ties. The Oedipus complex had sociological origins, arising from the frustration of man's wishes to be independent of patriarchal or authoritarian social arrangements.

Organized religion was a neurotic but generally accepted form of devotion and orientation, while neuroses were a form of private religion lacking patterned characteristics.

Social processes created anxiety, but the energies used in anxiety could be redirected into productive forces by social forces. Religious psychologists saw great possibilities for religion to act as the catalyst in eliminating this type of anxiety, because religion provided an orientation for man.

The fully developed personality was a combination of inborn endowments, early experiences in the family, and later experiences in a social group, which enabled people to relate to people and things, and to enjoy good object relations as an adult. He could work fruitfully, love others, and enjoy a satisfying religious life.

All object relations were symbiotic, leading to self-aggrandizement rather than the furtherance of an ideal. Throughout his life, man looked for a sense of unity and meaning, by progressing or by regressing, while he was frightened by his awareness of his separateness and loneliness. In the ultimate state of regression, man became a completely nonreflective animal. He was then free of his problems of awareness.

Fromm felt that the role of the analyst was a more active one than that assumed by Freud, although he used many Freudian techniques and accepted much of Freudian analytic theory. Fromm said that the analytic relationship was reciprocal. The analyst responded to the patient's communications according to what the analyst saw and felt, while trying to arrive at the patient's unconscious processes as they were operating at the time. The aim of treatment was increased responsibility on the part of the patient.

American theologians were most interested in the theories of Horney, Sullivan and Fromm, because they dealt with the contemporary problems of anxiety, loneliness and alienation. They also emphasized the role which the environment, of which religion in America was an important part, played in the cure of neuroses. Post–World War II psychologists recognized that irrespective of its absolute veracity, religion could be an integrating and supportive force in the life of the individual.

Social Scientists Discuss Religion

Before authorities in the field of religion could digest and react to Freudian psychology, social scientists and in particular psychologists had begun to study religion in terms of Freudian psychology. The first impact of this work was to widen the breach between social scientists and theologians, because the theologians suspected that many of these studies were designed to demonstrate the regressive and neurotic nature of religious practices and attitudes. The writings of psychoanalytic theorists like Freud, Rank, and Jung on the nature of religious belief and practices, the work of their followers on religious leaders and religious rituals, and the systematic attitude-testing which suggested that relationships existed between religious orthodoxy and bigotry, served to delay the acceptance of the mental health role of Freudian psychology by religious leaders.

An early example of the analysis of religious ritual in psychoanalytic terms was a study published by Jacob A. Arlow in 1927. He interpreted the Jewish practice of *bar mitzvah* in terms of the moral and sexual conflict that existed between father and son. Arlow thought that the *bar mitzvah* was a symbolic castration, and a resolution of the Oedipus conflict. In addition, he alleged that there was a correlation between the anxiety experienced by students before examinations, and the unresolved anxiety which remained from the *bar mitzvah* ritual.[1]

Psychoanalysts also studied primitive religions. Rôheim examined the religious practices of central Australian aborigines in 1932 in the light of psychoanalytic concepts. He said that soul of man was given a phallic personification by the aborigines who projected their superego onto ghosts. Rôheim felt that the concept of the soul was a projection of both the life and death instincts, and that the aboriginal view of paradise was sexual, and complete with funerary symbols of coitus.[2]

During the 1930s, anthropologists tested Freudian theories about the universality of the Oedipus complex among primitive people. They concluded from their field work that personality was the result of acculturation of instinctual drives. Interpersonal relations were more important than instinctual drives in determining personality, and sexual behavior was an outgrowth of personality, instead of the reverse.[3]

However, the displacement of sexual drives by culture was seen as the dynamic force in human behavior. This made it much easier for theologians to examine other psychoanalytic concepts to determine whether any could improve their "cure of souls." In this way the field work of anthropologists actually aided the acceptance of Freudian and neo-Freudian psychology by the theologians.

Modern Christianity was not immune to the scrutiny of social scientists. J. B. Holt conjectured that the "holiness sects" in modern Christianity represented an attempt on the part of the members to recapture security lost by too rapid migration.[4] Psychologists also examined the relationship of a minister to his congregation. E. M. Rosenzweig thought that ministers served as surrogate fathers to their congregations, and thus provoked conflicting emotions among congregants. When they were viewed as loving fathers, they encouraged feelings of affection; when they were hostile, they had the effect of a superego surrounded by taboos.[5]

Psychologists analyzed saints. J. M. Mecklin said that medieval saints were a product of their environment, not of divine grace. Local conditions and forces had changed in modern times, and saintly virtues were now discredited.[6] Hans Sachs analyzed St. Paul in terms of his struggle with strict control of his ego, while seeking freedom of the spirit. Sachs proposed that St. Paul was trying to reconcile the conflict between freedom and control, between life and death, and between the ego and the superego. St. Paul felt threatened by his desires, which would interfere with his constricted inner life; he reacted by equating sin with death. Specifically, St. Paul viewed that crucified Jewish messiah as the resurrected God of the contemporary mystery religions. Love to St. Paul meant identification with Jesus, and enternal life was gained through Jesus's death, which was the triumph of love and of life. Through death, it was possible to conquer sin.[7]

Some social scientists predicted that western civilization was about to enter a post-Christian era, in which the liberating concepts of psychoanalysis would be substituted for the "magical manipulations" of religion formerly used by man to free himself from guilt.[8]

Mysticism was a religious phenomenon which lent itself readily to psychoanalytic study. Herbert Moller examined effective mysticism, suggesting that the mystical state was made up of many fantasies and feelings which were involved in a vast defensive system in which God lost his masculinity and Jesus became the lover and father figure. He said that mysticism had declined in modern times, because of the sexualization of religion and the increased emphasis placed by society on mastery of the physical environment and the familial relations.[9]

Psychologists also studied correlations between religious and social attitudes, such as the relationship between authoritarianism and fundamentalism[10] or the relationship between religion, guilt, and ethics.[11] Some of these studies attempted to show that religious beliefs had a positive correlation with socially regressive attitudes,[12] while others sought to apply scientific principles to the study of religion.[13]

Much of this literature antagonized religious readers. Fortunately, there was some support for the acceptance of psychoanalytic concepts, mostly from hospital chaplains of all faiths.

Deeply involved in daily ministrations to their congregations, most ministers or institutional chaplains had little time for intellectual pursuits. Therefore, the impact of the studies was limited to those ministers who had the time and interest to read the learned journals in which they appeared.

V

Protestants and Psychological Theory

In the 1950s, after the shock of World War II, Protestant clergymen in large numbers embraced Freudian and neo-Freudian psychology. It was a decade or more after the death of Freud when this rapprochement occurred. The new interest in Freudian psychology was stimulated by the horrors of the Holocaust and the terrors of Communism. Wartime chaplains had felt deeply frustrated by their inability to abate battle-related neuroses and psychoses through traditional means. Feeling the existence of a need which they were unable to fulfill, ministers and chaplains began to investigate the new psychoanalytic concepts about the workings of the human mind and the existence of the unconscious. Those who had served as armed forces chaplains had received at least some training in psychoanalytic concepts and techniques as part of the training program for military chaplains.

Upon returning to civilian life, former military chaplains were pursuing their new interest in psychology. Some returned to school to study psychology, while others subscribed to newly founded journals like the *Journal of Pastoral Care*, the *Journal of Clinical Pastoral Work* and *Pastoral Psychology* when they assumed congregational or institutional ministries.

These journals linked the average minister seeking to apply the insights of psychology to his pastoral work with the theological seminaries where clinically trained ministers were teaching courses in pastoral counseling. Professors of pastoral psychology were the most frequent contributors to the journals of psychology and religion. Prominent neo-Freudians like Carl Jung, Karen Horney, Erich Fromm and Carl Rogers also contributed, as did social scientists like Margaret Mead. By subscribing to these journals, the average minister was able to learn of courses and seminars through which he could receive clinical pastoral training, of new literature relating to pastoral psychology, and of the thoughts of psychologists and eminent pastoral counselors who contributed to the journals.

Some of the new professors of pastoral psychology were experienced, clinically trained, institutional chaplains who had brought psychologically oriented pastoral care to the inmates of hospitals and prisons. Anton T. Boisen, Philip A. Guiles, and Russell C. Dicks were frequent journal contributors who often wrote of their experiences as institutional chaplains. Other professors, such as Seward Hiltner and Wayne E. Oates, were more concerned with the parish ministry, while others like Paul Tillich were most interested in the philosphical synthesis of psychology and religion. Occupants of prominent pulpits like John Sutherland Bonnell were frequent contributors, as were psychiatrists and psychologists who were interested in the application of psychoanalytic concepts to religion. Karl and William C. Menninger, Luther E. Woodward and Lawrence S. Kubic belonged to the latter group. The journals were interdenominational, although the more liberal Protestant denominations such as the Presbyterians and the Methodists were heavily represented, and *Pastoral Psychology* was proud to publish articles by interested Catholic and Jewish clergymen. It became the most widely consulted journal dealing with psychology and religion.

Pre –World War II

The delay in acceptance can be attributed to Freud's atheism, and to his emphasis on the role of the instincts and sexual drives. Early indications of a rapprochement were evident in the periodical press even before 1950. In 1928, an article appeared in *Mental Hygiene*, a publication which was more devoted to mental health than to religion, in which the author claimed that both the behaviorist psychology of Watson and the analytic psychology of Freud offered insights into man's behavior which could improve religious life. He further asserted that psychology could "illuminate the dark areas of character" and free the individual from his immediate concerns. Psychology could thereby enable laymen to feel more secure and happy and more receptive towards the joys of religious life.[1]

Two years later another article appeared in *Religious Education* to the effect that a mentally ill Christian might regain the soul which he had lost in the course of mental illness by means of the aid of psychoanalytic therapy employed by the churchmen.[2] Anton T. Boisen, the pioneer in the field of clinical training in psychology for ministers, published an important book in 1936 in which he said that religious workers could be helpful in the cure of the insane. He said that the insane experienced a period of crisis, in which religious faith could help them achieve a reorganization of their personalities. This reorganization after a conversion experience might be called recovery. Boisen felt that religious workers who were trained in psychology could enable the mentally ill to find health through Christianity.[3]

In 1940 an article published in *Mental Hygiene Review* emphasized that both religion and mental hygiene worked to build stable personalities. Therefore, a basis for cooperation between the two existed.[4]

At this same time, Seward Hiltner, later to be one of the leaders in the field of pastoral psychology, began to show an interest in the role religion could play in mental health. Hiltner suggested that religion could help a person integrate his whole life, if it were to be related to the entire personality in a noncompulsive and socially oriented way. Religion could help a person mature. Hiltner believed that clergymen should work with mental health workers.[5] The need for a healthy, well-integrated personality structure was one of his most frequently mentioned themes.

In 1943, K. R. Stolz published a monograph entitled *The Church and Psychotherapy,*[6] in which he discussed ways in which religious practices anticipated psychotherapy. While noting that the fellowship offered by the church could be of aid in the cure and in the prevention of neuroses, he warned that religion could not deal effectively with psychoses. He was also concerned about the "vocational neuroses" of clergymen. Fellowship was often cited as a great aid in the establishment and maintenance of mental health. Social isolation, where the furtherance of object relations was impossible, was recognized very early as one of greatest social problems.

1945–1950

In 1946, C. P. Landis theorized in the *Review of Religion* that psychotherapy was really central to the idea of pastoral care, and that pastoral care would be more effective if the new insights offered by psychology were utilized. He lamented the intransigence religious leaders had displayed towards psychology, and blamed this on the dogmatism of both religious leaders and psychologists.[7]

The *Journal of Pastoral Care*, published for the first time in 1947, provided a forum for religious workers who were convinced by the horrifying events of World War II that there was a great need for cooperation between those working in the fields of psychiatry and of religion. In its opening editorial, the *Journal of Pastoral Care* announced its intention to publish articles and other material which would otherwise not be easily available to pastoral counselors.[8]

An important article by David Roberts called "Theological and Psychiatric Interpretations of Human Nature" appeared in that first issue.[9] Accepting the existence of Freudian neuroses, Roberts contended that sin was the result of alienation from God, and that the alienated sinner could not effectively use his free will. Thus he removed sinners from the ranks of the evil, and placed them among the sick. Therefore, Christian ministers could be selective in their acceptance of psychoanalytic concepts, utilizing those which were helpful, and rejecting those which conflicted with their beliefs. On the other hand, he felt that a psychoanalyst could empoy a patient's religious faith as a tool in healing, without the psychoanalyst's having to accept that faith himself.

Roberts recognized that it was hard to develop dependence on God and responsibility for one's actions at the same time. He explained that self-pride was really a mask for self-rejection and therefore a prideful person should be viewed as an unhappy rather than a sinful person. The recognition of sin was important to religious leaders because it was considered to be the first step towards repentance and held possibility of religious conversion. He felt that the process of recognition of sin, repentance, and conversion might be likened somewhat to the psychotherapeutic process.

Roberts hoped for a fusion of psychoanalytic technique with religious beliefs, which he felt would be a great aid in the pastoral work of ministers. He recognized that much work had to precede such a synthesis. Some of the antipathy which psychiatrists often felt towards religion, he suggested, was really directed towards the authoritarian judgments made by religious leaders. Roberts urged that judgments of all people remain flexible. A more understanding and sympathetic attitude on the part of religious leaders towards neurotics and sinners would help the mentally ill assume greater responsibility for their actions and achieve active growth and maturity. Psychiatric experience indicated that condemnation was less effective than self-acceptance in encouraging growth in human relations. Roberts concluded that workers in the two fields should cooperate even though there were areas of disagreement which needed further exploration.

The Roberts article was an early synthesis of psychology and religion. Here were suggested ways in which the use of psychoanalytic concepts could help the pastoral counsellor prepare the client for a deeper religious life. In addition, Roberts fully recognized the problems in the way of full cooperation between psychology and religion.

Landis's earlier views on the importance of psychotherapy for pastoral counseling were reiterated in an article in the *Journal of Pastoral Care* in which he criticized ministers for not utilizing psychological insights in pastoral work. Landis warned the clergy that they were rapidly being shunted aside from their rightful place in American culture, because they had not adequately dealt with the problems of mental illness.[10]

Rollin J. Fairbanks, a prominent pastoral psychologist, made a plea in 1947 for cooperation between psychologists and the clergy. This cooperation was necessary, he said, for the welfare of all parishioners, and for patients in therapy in particular. He advocated prompt referrals between the types of healers, as soon as symptoms of any disorder were recognized. Fairbanks realized that much work was needed in order to develop a philosophical synthesis between psychology and religion and a program for sharing the management of specific cases.[11]

Albert Outler was another leader in the field of pastoral psychology who suggested a more limited acceptance of psychoanalytic concepts. In 1948, Outler supported assimilation of the practical wisdom of the mechanistic systems of psychology, but warned that Christian faith and theology had to be paramount at all times. Outler felt that man had a transcendental nature beyond Freudian formulations of the psychic system. Man was the possessor of free will, and was responsible for his actions. Therefore, the Christian counselor had to concentrate on the moral and spiritual attitudes of the client in an atmosphere of love, security, and the appreciation of the worth of the individual. Although Outler seemed to be interested in psychoanalysis, his basic concerns assumed acceptance of the traditional structure of moral responsibility.[12]

1950–1960

In the 1950s, a wave of books and articles appeared which called for cooperation between psychology and religion.[13] David E. Roberts published *Psychotherapy and a Christian View of Man*[14] in 1950. Roberts began by citing the wartime experiences of clergymen, especially those who served as chaplains in the armed forces, as proof that cooperation between psychology and religion was necessary. He declared that ministers who were not familiar with the concepts of psychology could not be effective pastoral counselors. Roberts denied that religion was in conflict with psychotherapy; more truthfully, religion and psychology were allies attempting to heal the sick. Roberts noted that the church could provide a powerful aid to the mental health community, because of the importance of religion in the United States. A man who was miserable because he was mentally ill could not experience Christian love and joy. Certainly, Roberts argued, the individual who attained the goals of maturity and responsibility through psychotherapy was an improvement over the conflict-ridden individual he had seen before. Arguing also that psychoanalytic concepts were useful in helping someone overcome grief and grow in the process, Roberts discovered a parallel between the Augustinian view of sin and the psychoanalytic concept of neuroses, for both depicted man as unable to change without outside help.

Thus Roberts tried to counter the arguments of those who said that psychology had nothing to offer religion, and bordered upon being an immoral philosophy, by the dictum that psychology was essentially moral. Wartime experiences had proven that psychology and religion could work in a partnership which was beneficial to mankind. Roberts used a full range of Freudian terms in his writings, and accepted the Freudian dynamic structure of the ego, the id, and the superego. He accepted Freud's theory of neuroses. He said that psychotherapy was moral because the goals of psychotherapy were human growth and the assumption of responsibility.

In the summer of 1950, Seward Hiltner, a pioneer in the advocacy of clinical training in psychology for ministers, discussed what he felt were the prime obstacles to the adoption of psychoanalytic techniques by religious workers.

Hiltner postulated that the life of an individual could only be understood in terms of dynamic forces, which included the forces of unconscious motivation. Only a person who was aware of the motives governing his behavior possessed the freedom to make the choices implicit in the operation of free will and the commission of sins. He cited dreams, slips of the tongue, and jokes as ways in which unconscious drives broke through to the conscious mind. Hiltner showed familiarity with Freud's *Psychopathology of Everyday Life*.[15]

Hiltner said that the mental life of man could only be known through developmental psychology, and that prior ways of thinking had to be abandoned in favor of this new knowledge. Some aspects of psychology were difficult to accept, especially the theories concerning infantile sexuality, penis envy among females, and the Oedipus complex. In addition, individuals might be resistant to learning about themselves. Hiltner urged that man could not know the truth from "conscience," "impulse," or "reason," but by combining the three, might attempt to find the truth. He concluded that psychology stressed the value of human life, shed new light on doctrines, and helped explain certain religious aberrations. Certainly the greatest good was the pursuit of truth, and the greatest evil was anything that caused deviation from the truth. Freud deserved credit for opposing what Hiltner called the "idolatrous ways" of religion, by which he meant the overemphasis on doctrine and ritual.[16]

The periodical *Pastoral Psychology* was first published in 1950. This journal offered a platform for discussions about the relationship of religion and psychology, and at the same time was a vehicle for the dissemination of information about the practical uses of psychology in the parish ministry in general, and in pastoral counseling in particular.

In an article in 1950, Lawrence S. Kubic stressed the importance of the patient's willingness to accept the integrity of the analyst, and to face unpleasant things about himself. Kubic noted that respect for the analyst was required, but not the blind faith found in faith healing.[17] Thus, once again, the importance of respect between therapist and client was stressed. The assumption was that although the therapist might not share the same religious convictions as the patient, love and acceptance were necessary for the development of object relations among all people.

In 1950, Lloyd E. Foster stated unequivocally in *Pastoral Psychology* that a pastor had to understand psychology in order to counsel; however, he still feared the effect of atheistic counselors upon the beliefs of religious patients. Some of the obstacles in the way of cooperation between psychology and religion included the rigid theological views of some of the ministers, coupled with their fears that the lifting of repressions of the sexual instincts would lead to sexual promiscuity. Ministers also resented Freud's labeling of religion as infantile, while they feared that psychology might replace religion as a system of belief. In closing, Foster cautioned that a therapist holding hostile feelings towards religion would probably transmit these views to his clients. Therefore, ministers should not refer patients for psychoanalytic therapy to anti-religious psychiatrists.[18]

Pastoral Psychology included a "Consultation Clinic"[19] where psychologically oriented ministers and psychologists tried to answer specific questions raised by ministers engaged in pastoral work, and offer solutions to problems. One important question was raised in the first year: namely, what moral stand could the minister expect the psychoanalyst to assume. The answer, given by both William C. Menninger of Menninger Clinic and by Seward Hiltner, was that the minister could not expect the psychiatrist to espouse any moral code, nor to be judgmental. The minister could, however, expect the psychiatrist to show good judgment, and to help the patient grow and be better able to make his own decisions. Ministerial concerns about the moral outcome of psychotherapy were only partially laid to rest by this answer. However, ministers were reassured that psychotherapists were indeed moral men who were little concerned with the morality eventually adopted by their patients.

Wayne Oates reviewed a book by Oskar Pfister entitled *Christianity and Fear* in 1950.[20] Pfister was a Swiss Protestant minister who, while not always in complete agreement with Freud, remained in friendly correspondence with him and accepted many of his theories.

In his review Oates stressed the importance of love in combating fear, and explained that Pfister's theory was based on Freudian psychology. The theory stated that a religion which created fears had to use magic, superstition, and ritual to combat fear. Thus, religious rituals resembled private rituals, which were obsessional or compulsive neuroses. By joining a religion, and trading his freedom and individuality for relief from tension, the individual could resolve his fears and compulsions. Pfister called a religion which substituted the observance of ritual for the seeking of inner peace neurotic religion. He said that the acceptance of religious truths depended upon the individual's attitude, which was based upon his inner needs and resulted from his life experiences. Pfister noted that Jesus resolved fears by love of God, but fear and repressions were reintroduced by St. Paul, the Roman Catholic Church, and the Protestant reformers of the Reformation. Pfister advocated the use of Christian love to eliminate fear.

The change in emphasis from acting out of fear to acting out of love was one of the most fundamental changes in theology caused by the acceptance of Freudian concepts. It occurred because theologians realized that religious growth could only occur through the furtherance of good object relations, and that they had to follow a pattern of self-love and acceptance, which could be followed by acceptance of others and lead to acceptance of God.

Paul Luschermer suggested that the inability to assume responsibility in church organizations, according to the theories of Karen Horney, might be another sign of neurosis. Horney said that a neurotic person thought in terms of fault and of punishment, and, therefore, found the assumption of responsibility difficult. She defined neurosis as self-alienation, accompanied by a decreased capacity for self-expression. Luschermer also mentioned the possibility of a neurotic whose feelings of responsibility were weakened by trying to hide them by over-compensation. He accepted Horney's definition of neurosis as a conflict between human instincts and cultural and environmental influences.[21]

The Menninger brothers, both of whom were psychiatrists, were prolific writers in the field of psychology of religion. Karl Menninger said in 1951 that hymns had therapeutic value, because singing hymns reduced anxiety and guilt and encouraged fellowship. He said that the new psychoanalytic concepts, particularly that of unconscious motivation, made it easier to understand and to cure mental illness. Psychoanalysis should not remove a sense of sin, which was really a theological matter, but psychology could deal with false guilt, which was a mental health problem. Thus, he differentiated between real and false guilt and sin. He further tried to reassure his readers that reports of sexual promiscuity among former psychoanalytic patients were exaggerated. What was labelled as promiscuity was really the emergence of normal sexuality among those in whom it had previously been neurotically suppressed.[22]

Seward Hiltner continued his advocacy of the acceptance of Freudian psychology as part of pastoral psychology in 1952. He now proposed that the initial response of churchmen to Freud's concept of the unconscious was negative because they feared that the acceptance of the concept of unconscious motivation would foster immorality. It was possible, he said, to accept Freudian concepts without accepting Freudian beliefs, and different psychologies should not be judged according to their acceptance or rejection of religion. A psychology should be judged by its effectiveness in helping a minister in his pastoral work.[23]

Also in 1952, T. J. Bingham explained why the Freudian concept of unconscious motivation posed a particular problem for Protestant theologians. He noted that Protestantism had eliminated the sacrament of confession, and made every man responsible for his own salvation. But the acceptance of the concept of unconscious motivation meant that man could not be held completely responsible for his own salvation. In addition, the difference in ethical standards in psychoanalytic practice and in church doctrine caused concern among ministers. Bingham advocated a merging of psychoanalytic insights with Christian ethics and philosophy as the solution to the conflicts between psychology and religion.[24]

Rollo May, a minister who was also an existentialist psychoanalyst, criticized Freud's labeling of all religion as compulsive neuroses. Some religions could be considered to be compulsive neuroses, May believed, while others could not. The distinction should be made according to whether or not the religion strengthened the dignity of the individual, gave him a feeling of self-worth, and increased his ability to make mature ethical judgments.[25] This emphasis placed on individual growth and maturity through religious maturity, rather than religious ritual, was an important change which showed the influence of psychoanalytic concepts on theology.

Albert Outler tried to reconcile psychotherapy with Christianity in a book entitled *Psychotherapy and the Christian Message*[26] in 1954. Outler accepted psychotherapy as a "healing art" while he tried to retain a Christian religious perspective. He said that psychology showed a genuine respect for the patient. Psychotherapy fostered growth and development, and when experienced with a Christian counselor, could lead to increased maturity without the necessity of moralizing by the therapist. Outler said that psychology had shown the importance of self-esteem, and Christian philosophy viewed the "human self" as "singular, substantial and responsible."[27]   When therapy ended man's estrangement from himself, he could then consider his estrangement from God.[28]   Man, he said, retained the responsibility for controlling impulses and directing them into channels considered moral by Christianity.[29]

Outler's position was that the concepts of psychotherapy had to be used against a backdrop of philosophy which was derived from the Gospels, and which reflected the ultimate meaning of life.   Psychotherapy could make a man sane, but only faith could free him from anxiety.   A Christian context for psychotherapy would "exalt man as his own savior."[30]   Outler agreed that psychotherapy had proven neurotic behavior meaningful.   Thus, Outler acknowledged the contribution of psychology to the cure of the mentally ill, and to an improved understanding of the aspects of Christian religious practice which best encouraged mature growth toward God, and the acceptance of Christianity.

In keeping with the emphasis on the encouragement of loving relationships, W. Bonaro Overstreet in 1953 stressed the importance of not allowing unloving people to fashion the church in their image.   He suggested that those who could only be receivers or takers in human relationships should be referred to medical help if admonitions and counseling failed.[31]

Roy A. Burkhart, in 1954, was concerned about the authoritarian attitudes which he found in his church.   He felt that his relationship to the church, including its governing boards, was essentially authoritarian. He was especially concerned that the ministry to the sick was authoritarian.   He thought that a healing ministry of fellowship to the sick might be more effective in fostering growth.[32]

In 1955, Carl Binger, a psychoanalyst, stressed the morality of Freudian psychoanalysis.   He said that it utilized the scientific method, which was by its very nature nonjudgmental, but the purpose of the analysis was to free the ego so that it could exercise responsible freedom of choice.[33]

A. Graham in 1954 showed the clear influence of Jung.   The author stated that all neuroses in people over age of thirty-five were fundamentally religious problems.[34]

Wayne E. Oates, another leader in the field of clinical training for ministers, rejected Freud's description of religion as an illusion.   He said that religion among the mentally ill and among primitive people might indeed be authoritarian and resemble a distortion of the parent-child relationship.   However, religion based upon Biblical prophecy and the teachings of Jesus Christ, as practiced by mentally healthy people, did not fit Freud's definition of religion as a neurosis.[35]

Thus Oates tried to show that although Freud's definition of religion did not accurately reflect Christian theology or practice, it was not entirely unfounded. On the whole, *Pastoral Psychology* gave marked impulse to the Freudian influence upon the Protestant ministry.

In 1956, Carroll A. Wise suggested that the Bible had anticipated certain psychoanalytic concepts, and was an aid to people suffering from normal guilt and anxiety. He defined anxiety as a state of tension which constituted a threat to the self. People who were capable of basic trust of faith, he felt, could find relief from anxious feelings by reading the Bible; Jesus had shown the reality of sin and the existence of real guilt with the accompanying states of estrangement and isolation. Wise discussed the development of a conscience and a sense of guilt in a growing child, and then differentiated between real and neurotic guilt. He said that Jesus also realized that forgiveness was the equivalent of love and of acceptance, which were prerequisites for mental health. Wise thought that a mentally ill man was incapable of loving. Jesus had also recognized the value of confession coupled with repentence and the fact that those who were filled with hatred were self-destructive. Noting the similarity between religious faith and the faith the patient had to have in the therapist in order for therapy to be successful, Wise declared it was the job of the pastor acting as a therapist to heal broken human relationships, using the techniques of psychotherapy which paralleled Jesus's teaching and retained a Christian theological framework.[36]

Wise tried to show that psychoanalytic concepts were in agreement with Jesus's teachings about the nature of man and human need, and thus to make psychoanalytic concepts more readily acceptable to ministers.

Seward Hiltner discussed the relationship between Freud, psychoanalysis and religion in an article with that title in 1956. He began by assuming that religion and psychology were not the same, although they could work together in a Christian context. Hiltner partially excused Freud's anti-religious statements by saying that Freud was dealing with aspects of infantile religion. But Freud could be justifiably criticized for ignoring ethical and moral aspects of religion. Hiltner believed, of course, that Freudian psychology had been criticized in the postwar era on religious and moral grounds, and attempts had been made to distinguish between Freud's theories and the theories of neo-Freudians such as Karen Horney. Hiltner noted that it was logically impossible to reject Freud's work while accepting the work of his followers, such as Jung, Adler and Horney, all of whom claimed that they had deviated from orthodox Freudianism. Deviation should not be confused with abandonment. Religious writers had to be selective in their criticism of Freud. Hiltner concluded that religion was concerned with man's "ultimate dimension." It was possible that psychological theories could help man achieve that dimension.[37]

Some pastoral psychologists preferred the theories of the neo-Freudian theorists such as Karen Horney, Harry Sullivan, and Erich Fromm to the theories of Freud, because the neo-Freudians de-emphasized the importance of the sexual instinct in the determination of human behavior.

Instead, the neo-Freudians stressed the importance of social factors in neuroses. Horney defined neurotic conflict in terms of moving from or towards people. Sullivan and Horney considered neuroses to be character disorders which required retraining, sometimes of a moral nature. The neo-Freudians were optimistic that, through retraining, patients could fulfill their potentials. Theirs was a philosophy which was easily compatible with traditional American optimism about the ability of people and conditions to improve. Protestant churches, with their numerous voluntary fellowship organizations, had vehicles which were well suited to encouraging supportive and loving retraining.

Carrol Murphy in 1957 wrote about the important of love and acceptance in counseling. He said that the therapist helped the client accept himself, by showing that the therapist accepted the patient. Self acceptance then acceptance of others would follow. Through acceptance, the patient could feel God's forgiveness and Christian love, which would help the patient heal himself.

Murphy agreed with Sullivan[38] that a person had areas of selective inattention. He agreed that unconscious material had to be made conscious, as Jung and Freud had stated. Murphy said that unconscious material became conscious in disguise, until the conscious mind was ready to deal with it openly. This was a reference to Freud's theory expressed in the *Psychopathology of Everyday Life.* Murphy was afraid, however, that when a therapist interpreted a patient's dreams, he was likely to "project" his own interpretation onto them.[39]

1960–1965

Protestant writers showed new sophistication in dealing with psychology in the 1960s. Obviously the battle for acceptance of psychoanalytic concepts in pastoral work had been won. For the first time, retrospective articles about the acceptance of Freudian psychology appeared in the journals of religion. The writers displayed considerable mastery of concepts of interpersonal relations of the neo-Freudians.

Revel L. Howe suggested some of the reasons for the acceptance of psychoanalytic concepts in pastoral psychology. First was the decline of late nineteenth-century liberal optimism in the face of the World Wars, and the deterioration of Catholic revival into ritualism. Filling this vacuum, the new insights of existentialist philosophy, and of Bible study, had shown man alienated from God, and in need of reconciliation with him. Therefore, the techniques of clinical psychology were utilized by pastors to meet modern needs for reconciliation, love and the surcease of anxiety.[40]

Leon Salzman, a Jewish psychiatrist, published an article in 1962 which asserted that the morality of the psychoanalytic process was in conformity with Judeo-Christian ethics.

Salzman believed that psychoanalysis, as developed by Freud and by the neo-Freudians, was moral, and concerned with man's moral existence. The cure of neuroses freed man from compulsions, which then enabled him to make free moral choices. Salzman noted that a person who was a compulsive neurotic might appear to be a very moral person, and it might be difficult to distinguish the moral from the neurotic.[41]

James A. Knight, a doctor who was active in the Protestant clinical training movement, discussed the similarities between Freud and Calvin, in an attempt to make Freud seem to be more like religious leaders than he probably was. He said that both were ascetic, although Freud believed the aim of sexual activity was the pursuit of pleasure, while Calvin held that sexual activity was only justifiable for procreation. Both were compulsive in their work habits. Calvin and Freud both said that man was not free. Calvin thought that man was depraved as the result of original sin, while Freud said that man labored under the domination of the id. Knight noted that both men were unforgiving in the face of what they considered heresy.[42]

One of the recurring themes in articles about the changes in pastoral theology caused by the acceptance of modern psychology was the emphasis on the need for man to have a group environment offering fellowship in which he could grow. Isolation was seen as the ultimate evil.[43] Another important theme was the importance of wholeness of the personality, which was seen as a reaffirmation of Biblical wholeness.[44] The great majority of articles emphasized the importance of sharing and cooperation between psychologists and theologians.[45]

The Acceptance of Existentialist Psychology
by Protestant Pastoral Psychologists

During the post–World War II decades, existentialism proved to be very compatible with Freudian approaches. Existential psychotherapy was attractive to certain theologians who were trying to formulate a psychology of religion. Existential philosophers were concerned with problems of anxiety, reason, freedom, values, authenticity, object relations, death, and most of all, the uniqueness of human existence.[46] Existentialist theologians, like Paul Tillich, shared their concerns and, in addition, wrote about the problems caused by man's finitude anxiety, his need for salvation, and a relationship with the divine. Existential psychologists, like Carl Rogers, Rollo May and O. Hobart Mowrer, utilized the concepts of Freud and the neo-Freudians in combination with the philosophical concerns of existentialism. Problems of anxiety, freedom of choice, will, and man's finitude had always concerned those trying to accommodate psychology and religion. Ideas unique to existentialist psychology included a disbelief that the past could ever accurately be related or reconstructed, and an interest in the effect of future plans and goals on the outcome of therapy. In addition, there was an emphasis on the conscious rather than the unconscious mind, and on action rather than discussion during the course of therapy. The emphasis on the conscious mind, action, and the future, was much more similar to the philosophy of traditional pastoral counseling than to orthodox Freudian analysis.

Paul Tillich, the famous existentialist philosopher and Protestant theologian, who was born in Germany and immigrated to the United States in 1933, endorsed the relationship between psychoanalysis and existentialist theology in 1958. Tillich praised Freud for resurrecting the concept of the unconscious, and noted that psychoanalysis and existentialism shared a concern about man's "existentialist predicament," or the question of man's estranged existence. Existentialist psychology dealt with problems of existence faced by the healthy and by the sick, said Tillich, while depth or Freudian psychology was used solely to combat neuroses and psychoses. However, Tillich felt that Freud was not aware of man's existential problems.

One of the important ideas of existentialist psychology, according to Tillich, was the explanation of the fall of man from God's grace as a change from existential goodness to existential estrangement. Other concepts included a definition of sin as self-estrangement, of salvation as the process of making whole again, and of the rediscovery of the value of counseling and of confession. Tillich also spoke of other elements in existentialist psychology which would not be acceptable to most other psychologists, such as the rediscovery of the demonic, and the existence of a reflection of the parent-child relationship in religion.[47]

In an article written two years later, in 1960, Tillich discussed the impact of pastoral psychology on theology. Pastoral psychology, he thought, dealt with man in both his "existential potentialities" and his "essential activities." But the widespread awareness of the existence of the unconscious mind had ended the old theological emphasis on free will. Modern psychotherapy had reintroduced the female element in Christianity, and emphasized the need for faith. Tillich concluded that the naturalistic philosophy with which Freud was familiar, in combination with idealism, formed the basis of existentialist philosophy. Thus he tried to bridge partially the gap between the existentialists and Freud.[48]

Carl Rogers, an existentialist psychotherapist with wide counseling experience, stressed the importance of providing the proper atmosphere for personal growth. He said that growth occurred when self-acceptance, awareness of one's effect upon others, sincerity, and mutual acceptance existed. Rogers expressed concern over what he considered the manipulative aspects of behaviorist psychologists, and the uses of projective psychological tests.[49] He was seconded by Paul Johnson, a prolific writer in the field of pastoral counseling, who praised Rogers for his work in the field. Johnson maintained that Rogers had demonstrated that directive counseling was not successful, because the patient developed resistance as the counselor tried to direct the therapy towards the therapist's goals. Johnson preferred what he termed "responsible counseling" in which both the counselor and the client set the goals of therapy together. Joint assumption of responsibility limited the amount of authoritarianism in the counseling situation.

Johnson felt that Rogers used counseling techniques which were developed by Rank. These techniques focused upon personal growth rather than on problems, and stressed emotional attitudes rather than intellectual formations. Rogers was more interested in the immediate situation than in the patient's history, and he tried to use the therapeutic experience to foster growth.[50]

Rollo May, then early in his career as a minister and an existentialist psychotherapist, asserted that the problem of our society was the failure to accept responsibility and to choose values which would enable man to integrate his personality. Religion and psychology both worked towards helping man integrate his personality by enabling him to resolve and understand socially-caused anxieties. May conceded that the concepts of Freudian psychology and of unconscious motivation in particular were necessary in order to understand the "depths of character" of modern man.[51]

He, unlike Niebuhr, stressed the worsening of man's social neuroses from the early twentieth century to the post–World War II era. During this period the sphere of man's self-estrangement had widened from the disassociation of sexual impulses from the self in the Victorian era, to total self-alienation and isolation after World War II. His viewpoint was that of a neo-Freudian who attributed the cause of neuroses to social, not biological, forces.

May discussed changes in the causes of guilt and anxiety feelings which had intensified conflict-ridden situations for man. He said that before World War I, when Freud was developing his early theories, individuals experienced great conflicts between the demand of Victorian sexual morality and the pressures of human instinctual needs. Victorian society demanded that people repress sexual feelings. This repression caused disunion of the personality structure of the individual, often accompanied by the appearance of hysterical symptoms.

May suggested that Rank had tied guilt feelings in the 1920s to feelings of inadequacy, self-consciousness, hyper-sensitivity and fear of responsibility. A new guilt-ridden, insecure, neurotic type had arisen by the 1920s.

The neurotic of the 1930s also experienced guilt, but as part of the general feeling of weakness, self-contempt, emptiness, and dependence noted by Karen Horney in describing the beginning of modern self-alienated man. He experienced conflicts between reason and emotion which May said were really conflicts between unconsciously held conflicting goals. This individual had not achieved selfhood, and was incapable of self-affirmation. His desires were reflections of his bourgeois culture and the precepts of his parents, which he continued to introject. Indications of alienation were vocational failure and resentment against society. Such a person had not established his own goals, but sought to please someone else, who assumed the role of his all-powerful parents. He needed to be directed, and often felt that he was being cheated. This dependent individual was still fighting his parents and was often attracted to totalitarian ideologies.

The problems of the post–World War II era were more serious than the problems of earlier eras, and more difficult to cure. They were character neuroses rooted in the inability of the individual to experience himself in his own right. Modern man found it difficult to experience his essential or existential existence.

The neurotic guilt feelings of the 1930s originated in man's guilt and shame about his dependence, and his vocational or economic failure. The man of the post–World War II era was less guilt-ridden because he was less well intergrated into his surroundings.[52]

The achievement of selfhood, or the re-affirmation of the self, was an important concern of existentialist psychologists. May defined the achievement of selfhood as the ability to release repressions, and to achieve a dynamic unity of conscious and unconscious desires which would make the person whole. Only through the achievement of selfhood could the individual experience satisfying human relationships in which he would be able to accept himself, authority, his own dependence, and autonomy at the same time. The new self-awareness achieved through selfhood would enable the individual to choose appropriate life goals. May said that psychoanalytic therapy might be necessary before selfhood could be achieved.[53]

In 1960 May added that healing through abreaction could take place through the use of symbols which were parts of myths which he regarded as part of man's transcendental capacity to go beyond the immediate situation into the "possible."[54] Thus he combined Jungian ideas about symbols and myths and the collective unconscious, and existentialist philosophy.

O. Hobart Mowrer, another prominent existentialist religious psychologist, also preferred the neo-Freudian to the Freudian definition of neuroses. Freud had pronounced that man's biological drives conflicted with the demands of civilization. Neo-Freudians, beginning with Fairbairn, developed a purely psychological formulation for the development of neuroses, emphasizing social and moral factors.[55] Mowrer concluded that real guilt existed and had to be accepted, in order for healing to occur.[56]

Charles Stinnette, another existentialist who was a Rogerian therapist, influenced by Jung as was May, thought that acceptance of the client and judgment of his actions could not be separated, because of the relationship that existed between thought and act. Stinnette said that the therapist's acceptance of the client paralleled God's acceptance of man through Christ. Stinnette differentiated between revelation and insight, saying that the achievement of insight was a human achievement, while revelation was a divine gift. He said that myths contained symbols which connected revelation and reason. Revelation existed on a continuum with reason, and provided the ultimate "gestalt" or understanding of the meaning of life. Stinnette noted that both theology and psychotherapy were integrative, and utilized man's capacity for "reflective action."

Psychology differed from theology because psychologists did not accept the doctrine of free will, but both psychology and theology believed that man had the capacity to change. Stinnette thought that Rogerian analysis, emphasizing phenomena, was a further development beyond Freudian analysis, which utilized free association.[57]

Stinnette's concerns were typically those of existentialist pastoral psychologists. He was concerned about placing therapy in a Christian context, about the relationship of thought and action, and about the acceptance and the analysis of phenomena which were a combination of things known or perceived through a combination of knowing and feeling.

Existentialist pastoral psychology was attractive to some ministers because it was a synthesis of psychoanalytic methods and Christian philosophy. Most clinically trained pastors, however, continued to utilize the neo-Freudian theories of Horney, Sullivan and Fromm, stressing the importance of object relations in an alliance with Christian philosophy.[58]

The Publication of Articles by Prominent Psychologists in Journals of Religion

Pastoral Psychology and the *Journal of Pastoral Care* continued to feature articles and reviews of books by prominent neo-Freudian psychologists and recommended the the works of neo-Freudians such as Karen Horney to their readers.[59]   This had the effect of making the newest developments in the field of psychotherapy immediately available to the readers.

It was in *Pastoral Psychology* that Karen Horney explained why she thought that "the drive for glory" and Adler's explanation of striving for superiority were really not indicative of a religious person. Horney said that the "drive for glory" revealed a lack of self-confidence which had begun as self-alienation. The self-alienation caused the person to try for self-glorification, and the lack of self-identity resulted in self-idealization. Self-glorification was a neurotic solution, and often involved a search for vindictive glory.

Horney regarded such striving of the ego as neurotic pride, which trapped people between the need to preserve the self system and neurotic symptoms. Freud had characterized the same type of neurotic striving as a conflict between the cohesive ego and the anarchic id. Horney said that self-hate was the underside of pride.[60]

The sympathetic attitudes of leading theologians toward neo-Freudian psychologists were exemplified by Reinhold Niebuhr's praise of Horney as a creative psychologist. He was particularly interested in her theory that undue self-assertion arose because of the insecurities found in a capitalistic culture. Niebuhr thought that psychiatry could eliminate undue self-assertion, and that Christian thought would be enriched by the insights of modern psychiatry. The "half truths" of Freudianism and of neo-Freudianism balanced the "half truths" of Christian thought.

Theologians were attracted to certain aspects of psychoanalytic theory while they showed hesitation about some ramifications. Niebuhr preferred Freud's biological view of man dominated by his instincts, which he called the "Freudian naturalistic version" of original sin. Not agreeing with the neo-Freudians, who attributed man's problems to social and historical causes, he worried about the effects of neo-Freudian theories upon society. He felt rather that the acceptance of Sullivan's theory of neuroses would cause people to spoil their children because they might be afraid that discipline of the children would lead to childhood neuroses. However, he called Sullivan "the most persuasive of the neo-Freudians," and attributed to him the theory that undue self-assertiveness was caused by lack of security in the period of the self's infancy. Niebuhr agreed with Sullivan that the capacity of love was drawn from the security developed during childhood. He suggested that this theory shifted the responsibility for an individual's undue assertiveness from himself to his mother.[61]

C. W. Morris, a psychiatrist, was concerned about the effect of the neurotic church member on church organization. He applied the theories of Karen Horney to show that a person who did many "good works" in a church organization might be exhibiting symptoms of neuroses which could be harmful to the organization. Morris said that although the person's work might be useful, he should be directed away from good works into activities which encouraged loving relationships, which were what he really needed. Morris believed that the four types of neuroses listed by Horney — submission, neurotic affection, power, and retreat into materialism — all offered protection against imagined harm.[62]

The theories of Erich Fromm were also of special interest to pastoral psychologists, because of his emphasis on the importance of interpersonal relations and on the role of culture in defining healthy behavior.[63] His books were favorably reviewed in the journals concerned with the psychology of religion to which he contributed articles. Seward Hiltner relied upon Fromm's theory of good or bad characters, to prove that "moral actions" depended upon character integration.[64]

The foremost existentialist theologian, Paul Tillich, reviewed *Psychoanalysis and Religion,* by Erich Fromm. Tillich suggested that Fromm's greatest interest in the study of religion was the determination of whether it encouraged love and the pursuit of truth among men. Fromm opposed authoritarian religion, which placed all goodness and power in God. He preferred a humanistic religion which centered around man and his strengths. Fromm thought that God should be viewed as a symbol of man's power. Fromm conceded that psychology and religion shared some interests, but had different goals.

Tillich's viewpoint differed from Fromm's. Tillich thought that psychology was the study of the soul, which could not be separated from ontological or existential questions. Tillich agreed with Fromm that the religious images developed by people were projections of images from childhood, which could be either healthy or unhealthy. He maintained, however, that these images bore no relation to the actual existence of God. He felt that any psychology of religion had to deal with the divine in man, which Tillich said could be dealt with as man's existential existence, or as the supernatural in man.

Tillich praised Fromm for his "self-transcending humanism," which he preferred to the prevalent theism. Tillich defined sin as a separation from one's essential being with its divine dimension. He said that salvation was achieved by "healing the split," or reunification of all parts of one's self to achieve a holistic state. This reunification could only be accomplished with God's transcendental power, which also gave man the ability to accept himself.[66]

Tillich was familiar with other neo-Freudians. He used Horney's theory of ego splitting and reunification to explain in dynamic terms the reorganization and the focusing of the entire human person on the achievement of a satisfying Christian experience.

As for Fromm himself, he compared the psychologies of Freud and of Jung in *Pastoral Psychology* in 1950. He insisted that questions about Freud's and Jung's views on religion could not be dismissed by saying that Freud was the enemy of religion, while Jung was the friend. Fromm noted that Freud had identified the core of ethical religion as brotherly love, the reduction of suffering, and the increased ability for independent and responsible action by the individual. Jung, though he seemed to be friendlier, actually had reduced religion to a psychological phenomenon, during which man submitted himself to an external power. Fromm concluded that in the submissive state, truth and moral responsibility were undermined.

As Fromm saw it, Freud had placed the origin of religion in man's anxiety in the face of his helplessness in the natural environment and in resisting the instinctual drives from within.[67] Man repressed those problems which defied rational solution by developing religious beliefs. The illusion of religion enabled man to regress to a childlike state, and to perform rituals which resembled obsessional neuroses in children.

According to Fromm, Freud rejected religion because it sanctified its allies regardless of their intrinsic merit. It also weakened the power of critical thought by denying its veracity in dealing with religion. Fromm said that religion thereby weakened reason. According to religious philosophy, ethics were rooted in religion, which left ethics on less than firm ground among those who were not religious. Therefore, it was necessary to reject the illusion of religion and fully utilize reason. Man had to learn to accept and live with his insignficance. But Jung had said that religious truths existed because many people believed in them. The veracity of religion was subjective. Therefore, Fromm accused Jung of reducing religion to an unconscious phenomenon and elevating the unconscious to a religious phenomenon.[68] Fromm claimed that religion had both a subjective and objective existence. The veracity of revelation or reason depended upon the attitude of society.

In this analysis of Freud's and Jung's theories of religion, Fromm's preference for Freud's theories was clear. Fromm's overriding concern was the development of a religion stressing human relationships and ethical conduct. Fromm felt that Freud's concerns about the nature of society were closer to his own than were Jung's.

Anton T. Boisen, who pioneered in the field of clinical training, disagreed with Fromm's definition of religion. Boisen said that Fromm and Freud characterized religious experience as fostering self-reliance and independence. Jung, according to Fromm, described a religion which was based upon dependence, and submission to a higher power. Boisen believed that the dependent relationship of the child to the parent was transferred through religious education to a dependent relationship between a mature person and God. Just as a child needed a parent, Boisen thought that an adult needed God. Thinking that social morality depended upon religious beliefs, he believed, as did Jung, that part of religion came from a collective unconscious, and held that some forms of insanity were religious phenomena which were also rooted in the unconscious.[69]

Erich Fromm offered a critique of Freud's philosophy in 1962, with a caution that psychology was not a substitute for religion. Fromm increasingly appreciated the role of religion in helping man relate to his environment, and thereby lessening his isolation and alienation. He said that, viewed as a system, Freud's philosophy was a blend of romanticism, rationalism, the philosophy of the Enlightenment, and an interest in mythology and the supernatural. Fromm explained that Freud emphasized the exploration of the unconscious mind because he believed man's freedom came from understanding and overcoming his unconscious drives. He reiterated that Freud's opposition to religion was really a plea for the primacy of truth.

As for Freud's views on sex, Fromm felt that they reflected the Victorian milieu in which he lived. Freud, therefore, denied the existence of female sexuality and attributed penis envy to all women. This attitude reflected the inferior position of women in Victorian society. Fromm considered that Freud was no libertine, but wished only for a moderate reform of Victorian attitudes towards sex.

Freud used the scientific method of observation and recording; his theories were not unfounded. Fromm characterized the Viennese as a pessimist who believed that the demands of culture and man's instinctual needs were irreconcilable, and hinted that some neo-Freudians were making revisions because it suited their self-interest. He characterized Adler's theory of man's drive for superiority as being typical of the attitude of the lower middle class in the 1920s and in the 1930s. He praised Jung for his deeper understanding of the symbolism of the unconscious.[70]

Carl Jung, one of Freud's early disciples, was nearing the end of a long and illustrious career. He, unlike Fromm, never seemed aware of postwar social changes. His works were also of great interest to pastoral psychologists, because Jung was the most prominent of the Christian psychoanalysts, and he had a special interest in religion and mythology. In 1956, Jung expressed astonishment that anyone but a clergyman should be consulted about spirtual suffering. He could not understand why any pastors utilized Freud's theories about sexuality or Adler's theory of power. Jung said that these theories were equally hostile towards spirituality, and charged that both Freudian and Adlerian analysts were treating patients whose main problem was their spiritual alienation. Jung suggested that neuroses developed more frequently when religious life declined. Disturbances in the conscious life reflected meaninglessness in the unconscious. Freudian analysis merely exposed the darkness in the individual without elucidating it. Jung expressed doubt that man could understand the meaning of unconscious material without help. The unconscious contained defense mechanisms consisting of age-old fantasies which appeared when the possibility of danger to the psyche existed.

The unconscious was inexhaustible, extending beyond the personality, Jung asserted. Religious life contained elements from the unconscious. Jung believed that churches interposed dogma between the individual and material from his unconscious mind, which might become conscious during dreams. The churches limited what Jung considered to be real religion, and these limitations resulted in the need for a variety of religions suitable to different people. Jung felt that religion was an integrative force which encouraged mental health.[71]

Jung's writings elicited comments from the readers of *Pastoral Psychology*. J. Maxwell Chamberlin complained that Jung's concept of incarnation was not Christian, and expressed "dismay" over Jung's denial of the veracity of the historical Jesus[72] and his concept of incarnation. Seward Hiltner agreed.[73]

Hiltner offered his own estimate of Jung's description of the soul, the unconscious, including the persona, the concept of anima and animus, and Jung's psychological topology.[74] Jung explained religion as a psychic occurrence in which myth expressed what was happening in the soul. Mythological characters were models of psychological types. The psyche contained both good and evil, although Jung said that western civilization ignored the evil. Perhaps Jung felt that the Trinity should include the devil! He thought that Catholicism changed psychic symbols into objects, while Protestantism replaced them in the psyche, enabling the process of "individuation" in religion to proceed.[75] Although Jung's theories might interest theologians, they were less attractive to pastoral psychologists, because they related less to the problems pastors encountered when counseling parishioners. The average pastor had to deal with people who were troubled by grief, anxiety, and loneliness. Neo-Freudian theories of interpersonal or object relations offered more pertinent suggestions for the cure of these sicknesses and the alleviation of neuroses than did Jung's theories. Other important psychologists contributed articles.

Clara Thompson, a noted psychologist, discussed a sensitive topic, the changing role of women, in 1953. She conjectured that Freud's theory of penis envy in women was indicative of the lower status of women in Victorian society, where women were relegated to the low-status job of homemaker. She noted that the economic and social status of women was now changing, since an increasing number of women were now employed outside the home, and in higher paying jobs than ever. Thompson declared that a new psychology of women was needed, to resolve the conflicts in times of rapid change.[76]

William Reich's psychoanalytic theories were discussed by Leon Salzman in the *Journal of Pastoral Care* in 1954, in an objective manner, although Reich's theories stressing the importance of orgasm were probably quite abhorrent to many ministers.[77] Salzman emphasized Reich's contributions in describing character disorders rather than just describing symptoms. He noted that Reich's work in the field of character analysis had been further developed by Horney and by Sullivan, and that Reich's later theories were less widely accepted.[78]

Seward Hiltner, a pastoral psychologist, reviewed the theories of Theodor Reik, which were of interest to pastoral psychologists because Reik separated sex and love.[79] Reik said that love was more important than sex, and that sexual perversions were not just sexual aberrations but aggressions which were turned upon a sexual object. According to Reik's theory Christian love, or *agape,* could once again be considered to be free of sexual overtones.[80]

Reik denied that neuroses had a sexual origin, and confined sexual satisfactions to those which resulted from the sex act. He said that the greatest ego need was the need for affection, which was felt by all young and old.

Reik's *Dogma and Compulsion* was reviewed for *Pastoral Psychology* by a psychiatrist, Walter Stokes. He declared Reik's theories showed a close parallel between the way in which an insecure child resolved family conflicts by adopting "unreal obsessively valued compromises," and the way in which religious dogma had arisen.[81] People used religious dogma to achieve the same kind of security that the child derived from his compromises. Strokes recommended Reik's book to all counselors who wished to try to understand the significance of irrational obsessive mechanisms in religious beliefs.

The Use of Psychological Terminology by Theological Writers

The use of psychological terminology in articles about pastoral psychology indicated not only acceptance of the new psychoanalytic concepts, but also sufficient familiarity with the terminology to use these concepts in writing. Some pastoral psychologists and ministers seemed to command the vocabularies of psychology and religion with almost equal ease.[82]

By 1965 many Protestants viewed aspects of the human condition in terms which had been first suggested by psychoanalysis. Led by professors of pastoral psychology like Hiltner, Outler, Johnson, Fairbanks, and Boisen, ministers generally acknowledged the importance of good object relations in the life of an individual, and that they preceded a healthy religiosity. Speaking of sinners as sick rather than evil people, who suffered from neuroses which were generally rooted in childhood experiences, ministers sought clinical training to learn to make pastoral counseling therapeutic.

As theologians separated psychoanalytic techniques from Freudian philosophy, they found that neo-Freudian psychoanalysts were increasingly appreciative of the role religion could play in lessening man's feelings of alienation and anxiety. Articles praising the role of religious beliefs and practices which stressed love appeared alongside those adapting psychoanalytic concepts and techniques to the problems of pastoral counseling. They were often written by leading neo-Freudians and appeared in the journals of psychology and religion. Existentialist theologians and psychologists attempted to formulate an existential pastoral psychology, but most pastoral psychologists simply accepted those psychoanalytic theories which best seemed to explain the problems of contemporary man and suggest ways in which organized religion could ameliorate man's psychological distress.

Catholics, Jews, and Psychological Theory

It was especially difficult for Catholics to reconcile orthodox Freudian psychology with Catholic or Thomistic philosophy or psychology, because according to Thomistic doctrine man's reason or rational mind was sovereign. Therefore, many Catholics were attracted by the neo-Freudian psychology of Horney, Fromm, and Sullivan, which said that neuroses originated from bad interpersonal or object relations, or from a bad self-image, all of which came from the environment, and were subject to environmental modifications. Traditionally, Catholics had assumed that the sacraments contained all the aids to mental health that were needed. Nor could they accept sexuality as the motivating drive in man; most believed that talking about sexual thoughts would lead to sexual arousal, which they considered immoral. Finally, Freud stressed the domination of the irrational, demanding, unconscious id, and denied the objective existence of God, which was the foremost tenet of Catholic belief.

In contrast to Protestantism, where pressure for the acceptance of psychoanalytic insights came first from chaplains in institutions, later from former military chaplains, and after World War II from the parish ministry, members of the American Catholic Philosophical Association were the leaders in the fight for acceptance of psychology. Although Catholic institutional chaplains and social workers did urge an early synthesis of psychology and religion, their appeals were voiced only in Catholic medical and social service journals, and never seemed to affect the wider audience of the parish ministry or of Catholic laymen.

E. W. Weir, a Catholic theologian, opened the philosophers' argument for acceptance of Freudian psychology in 1936. Suggesting that psychological theory should be taught apart from the philosophy of the psychologists, and with a background of Catholic philosphy, he sought to place psychoanalysis in a Catholic framework.[1] Partial acceptance of psychology would be the usual tactic of Catholics trying to reconcile psychology with religion.

Sister M. Jeannette, an educator, had already proposed a compromise between Freudian psychology and Catholicism in 1931. She postulated that free association was a useful tool to use in the treatment of neurotics, and agreed with Freud in stressing the importance of traumatic experiences in the development of neuroses. While disagreeing with Freud's emphasis on the sexual libido as the source of human energy, Sister Jeanette did comment that the search for immortality represented a desire to return to the womb.[2]

Requests for cooperation between people working in the fields of psychology and religion continued in the postwar era. Catholics in social welfare agencies were among the first to recognize that mentally ill people were unable to respond to the traditional ministrations of the church.[3] Yet, Abridge V. White voiced a general sentiment when he said that there had to be a place for religion within psychotherapy.[4] Robert P. Odenwald, who was later to attempt a Catholic synthesis of Catholicism and psychology, added that not everything about psychotherapy was unacceptable to a Catholic.[5]

The increase in mental illness caused by battlefront and home tensions during World War II, and the return to civilian life of clinically trained priests, caused an upsurge in interest in psychotherapy among Catholics. There seemed to be more mental illness than ever before. Many Catholics hoped that people working in the fields of psychology and religion could cooperate in a way that was acceptable to Catholics, although they were very unsure as to the nature of the synthesis which was required.

Harry McNeill declared in 1947 that cooperation between the Catholic church and psychologists was essential. Catholicism could offer a philosophy which would help unify the discipline of psychology, but Catholics would have to acknowledge the role of the unconscious in the mental life of man and the fact that psychologists had discovered techniques for dealing with the unconscious. Feeling that the church was not effectively dealing with problems of excessive guilt and problems of sexuality, he urged that traditional Catholic thought be modified according to the new insights of psychology.[6]

Some Catholics were willing to trust psychiatrists but not clinical psychologists, a new class of professionals who developed during World War II.[7] Many lamented the lack of Catholic psychiatrists and psychologists, and suggested that priests should receive training in psychology.[8] However, A. McDonough warned in 1949 that since the church had yet to take a position on the morality of psychoanalysis, Catholics should proceed with caution in their relations with the new discipline.[9]

William Boyd pronounced Adlerian psychology compatible with Christianity, because it stressed love and the role of the community in which the person lived, in providing a mentally healthy environment. He believed that the theories of Freud and Jung would never be compatible with Catholicism.[10]   Meanwhile, many writers continued to support cooperation between psychiatrists and priests.[11]   Behind their persistence was a rationale similar to R. P. Odenwald's explanation of the nature of the differences between Catholicism and psychology.[12]   Odenwald said that most Catholics objected to Freudian psychology.   In the field, however, Catholic psychiatrists used psychoanalytic techniques while rejecting materialistic Freudian "doctrine."   He concluded that psychoanalysis was acceptable when it was administered by a Christian.[13]

By the 1950s, increased contact made Catholics feel that most psychiatrists and psychologists would not give advice which would lead to immoral activity,[14] and a growing number of writers, almost all of whom were in religious life, showed an understanding of the role of psychiatry in the cure of the mentally ill.   For example, J. Rumaud thought that psychology offered many concepts necessary for the understanding of the mind.   Conceding the existence of the unconscious mind, he was concerned about how the theory of unconscious motivation would affect the belief of Catholics that an individual was morally responsible for his actions.   He felt that the priest and the psychiatrist should agree on guidelines, to help both to distinguish problems of morality from problems of mental illness.[15]   James VanderVeldt[16] also urged cooperation between psychiatry and religion.   He asserted that religious beliefs aided mental health, and only psychologists could cure the mentally ill. However, psychology was not a substitute for religion.[17]

In 1952, Pope Pius XII condemned the "pansexual" method of psychoanalysis.   He failed to designate other methods of psychotherapy, and many Catholics expressed the need for further guidance on the subject.   His statement seems to have had little effect upon most Catholic writers, who were clerics and who had already rejected Freud's theory about the sexual etiology of neuroses as being unacceptable to Catholics.[18]

The Guild of Catholic Psychiatrists was formed in 1952.[19]   The Guild first tried to identify those elements of psychology which were acceptable to a Catholic.   Karl Stern said in their *Bulletin* that the insights into the human mind offered by Jung and by Freud were beneficial when stripped of their materialistic philosophy.[20]   At this stage, Jung's ideas were attractive and convenient.   For instance, A. White said that psychology and religion could be reconciled if psychology stopped treating religion as an obsessional neurosis.   He noted that dogmatism on both sides had decreased, and that Jung's theories had directed the attention of psychologists to the importance of religious imagery in mental health.   Jung had shown man's need for religion.[21]

Among Catholic theologians, C. H. de Haas was one of the few to think that a synthesis of Catholicism and Jungian psychology was possible. He reviewed Jung's dream theory and Jung's theories about the structure of the collective and individual unconscious, agreeing with Jung's statement that every neurotic person over thirty-five years of age had a religious problem.[22]

Gregory Zilboorg, a convert to Catholicism and a psychoanalyst, was the foremost advocate of Freudian psychology among Catholic theologians. He asked in 1954 that Freud be judged on the basis of the success of his techniques, without considering his views about God.[23] Many other theologians tried to distinguish between Freudian psychology, techniques, and philosophy. They tried to achieve a synthesis of Catholic philosophy, Freudian techniques, and most of the elements of Freudian psychology.

In 1954, John C. Ford, a prominent Jesuit theologian, wrestled with the problem of whether a Catholic could be psychoanalyzed. He decided affirmatively, even though psychiatry and religion had radically different viewpoints, and explored different areas of human existence. Despite Freud's denial of man's free will and Freud's atheism, a Catholic could be psychoanalyzed. Ford conceded that sex could be mentioned in the course of a psychiatric interview, even though the sexual content of the unconscious mind which might be brought forth by free association might be sexually stimulating to the neurotic. Moral law was not violated unless the patient deliberately indulged himself in "unchaste" "fantasies," "emotions," and "desires."[24] Ford saw much that was praiseworthy in Freudian psychology. He said that while he really did not understand the process of free association or abreaction, he did consider Freudian psychology to be the most profound investigation of the non-spiritual elements of man's nature presently available.

Agostino Gemelli hoped to bypass one of the conflict areas between Freudian theory and religion by the assertion that modern psychologists no longer accepted the Freudian theory of the sexual instinct as the motivating force in man's mental life. Neo-Freudians especially did not make it central to the process of psychoanalysis. As a result, psychiatrists and priests were cooperating in many areas, including institutions where priests served as chaplains and in seminars.[25] Obviously Gemelli had a preference for the neo-Freudians.

Jacques Maritain, another convert who remained a layman, in 1956, like Zilboorg, tried to separate Freudian techniques and Freudian theory from Freudian philosophy. Maritain thought that Freud's psychoanalytic technique was a work of pure genius, and that his psychology was good, but he found Freud's materialistic philosophy unacceptable. Maritain agreed with Freud's theory about the structure and the role of the unconscious, and about the function of dreams. Religion needed psychology. The sacraments of religion such as confession could not cure neuroses.[26]

Another theologian, W. C. Bier, agreed that a Catholic could accept Freud's dynamic system of psychology, and reject his philosophy. He advised Catholic psychologists to realize that Freud's religious opinions reflected his personal problems; neurotic patients also used their religious beliefs in the service of their neuroses just as they used everything else. Bier suggested that neo-Freudian psychotherapists like Jung held views which were more acceptable to Catholics because neo-Freudians recognized the role religion played in promoting mental health. Therefore, a Catholic could accept Freud's clinical findings, and reject his philosophy.[27]

In 1958, Pope Pius XII condemned Freudian psychology. He said that there were parts of the human conscience which could not be explored, because it was immoral to reveal information which was received in confidence. It was also immoral to explore sexual impulses, because the exploration might lead to sexual excitation. Neither the patient nor the therapist could indulge in any action which contravened moral law, or sought to make the irrational parts of the human personality sovereign over reason. However, the Pope added that, within the limits of Catholic morality, psychotherapists and Catholics could cooperate.[28]

The Pope's statement on the limits of psychotherapy modified only slightly the positions taken in the public debate over acceptance. Odenwald and VanderVeldt had discussed the basic elements in their synthesis much earlier. The argument over what elements of Freudian psychology were acceptable, therefore, continued with minor changes. Significantly, the Pope did not prohibit further discussion.

Most pastoral psychologists, whether Protestant, Catholic, or Jewish, continued to prefer the theories of the neo-Freudians, especially Horney, Sullivan, and Fromm, which stressed the role of social over biological factors in the development of neuroses. Psychiatrists, however, tended to retain a more Freudian orientation.

James H. VanderVeldt and Robert P. Odenwald now tried to establish a definitive guide to psychiatry for Catholics in the light of the Pope's condemnation of Freudian psychology. First they discussed the nature of personality and the determinants of human behavior. Man's personality, they asserted, was formed by the interaction of his natural endowments with the environment. God had given man free will to choose right from wrong, and grace to help him choose the right way. But grace was not coercive and did not prevent man from sinning.

Divine grace could, however, produce dramatic changes in personality, as it had done in the cases of St. Paul and St. Augustine.[29] Odenwald and VanderVeldt stressed that Catholicism had long recognized the existence of mental illness. Psychic conditions could cause physical illness, and psychosomatic illness proved the validity of Catholic doctrine about the unity of mind and body.[30]

The authors next discussed types of treatment of mental illness. They declared that many types of mental illness could be cured by treating the symptoms and modifying the environment in which the person lived. Environmental therapy included play therapy, group therapy, and changes in the home situation. In the case of a devout narcissistic person, prayer could sometimes be effective, because of the strong autosuggestion it created.[31] At times reassurance could be very effective. Free association was an acceptable technique only if sexual topics and information received in confidentiality were excluded.[32]

Rejecting all aspects of Freudian philosophy and those Freudian theories which were derived from the Freudian view of the nature of man,[33] they accepted only those aspects of Freudian psychology which could be independently validated. However, the technique of depth therapy initiated by Freud was acceptable. In treating Freud's philosophy they identified his denial of the objective reality of God as one of the major obstacles to its acceptance by Catholics. Freud said that God had subjective reality because he existed in the minds of men, but Catholics had absolute and certain knowledge of God. In addition, Freud considered sex the motivating drive in man's life, while Catholics said that man was motivated first by love of God, and secondly by love of man, according to the rule of "love thy neighbor as thyself."

Another area of conflict was the Freudian theory that the motivating drives in human behavior were located in the unconscious mind. Catholic theology stated that the rational mind controlled human behavior. Pope Pius XII said that man could never escape responsibility for his sins even though he might be mentally disordered.

In summarizing the basis for cooperation between psychiatry and religion, Odenwald and VanderVeldt held that sincere religious convictions were an aid to mental health especially when personal conduct was based upon religious beliefs. Psychiatry and religion could not be substituted one for the other. Furthermore, it was difficult to compare them because religion dealt with the supernatural. There was no conflict between Catholicism and psychiatry as long as psychiatry did not violate any of the principles of Catholicism. They preferred neo-Freudian psychology because it de-emphasized the importance of the sexual urges and stressed the role of the environment. Undoubtedly, neo-Freudian psychology presented fewer problems for Catholicism. As long as the psychotherapists did not encourage the patient to commit an immoral action, neo-Freudian therapy was acceptable and deemed necessary for the cure of mental ills.[34]

J. V. Abearonla soon raised some moral problems involved in the practice of psychotherapy, which had also been foreseen by Odenwald and VanderVeldt. He asked what was to be done when the patient was aware of his moral problems, but could not control himself enough to hold back from continuing to sin. Abearonla agreed that ego psychology was more compatible with Catholicism than was the psychology of the unconscious.[35]

Catholics were never able to resolve the problem of how free will operated in a mentally ill person. One solution was to argue that sin was only in proportion to the degree of understanding which the individual possessed. By this logic, mortal sin was impossible when a neurosis or psychosis inhibited reason.[36]

Practitioners continued to find Freudian methods of analysis useful in curing some forms of mental illness. In order to try to make Freud more acceptable to Catholics, M. Steck showed similarities between Thomistic psychology and Freudian psychoanalysis. For example, St. Thomas looked to the universe and saw God, while Freud looked and saw nature. It was possible also to detect a substantial similarity between the Freudian id and St. Thomas's doctrine of sensuality. While the superego could not be equated with St. Thomas's concept of conscience, the functioning of the superego could reveal something about the functioning of a childish conscience. He concluded by stating that much of Thomistic and Freudian thought was similar, and that it was possible to learn from Freud.[37]

In 1958, Gregory Zilboorg modified his support of Freudian psychology, in the light of Pope Pius XII's condemnation. Zilboorg admitted that there were parts of man's conscience which could never be probed, nor could the priest reveal secrets entrusted to him in the confessional. He then called attention to the Pope's dictum that psychiatrists had to be moral men who were aware of the moral teaching of the Church, and his assurance added that clergymen and psychologists could cooperate.[38]

In the same year, Zilboorg focused upon Freud's attitude towards religion. He wrote that Freud's attitude reflected his personal problems, especially Freud's death wish theory. He concluded that Freud was interested in metaphysics, but hostile towards religion; Freud had never understood religion as it was understood by a believer.[39]

By the late 1950s, increased numbers of priests and psychologists were cooperating. Catholic writers took note of the fact, and tried to describe the nature of this cooperation. Marc Oraison, a cleric, explained in 1958 how psychoanalysts and priests could assist one another. Since a good psychiatrist refrained from all value judgments, said Oraison, the patient fell back upon his own values.

The priest could encourage mental health through judicious use of the sacrament of confession and forgiveness of sins, but he should discourage obsessional confessions.   He might be the object of transference neurosis. He should not stand between man and God, and he should be careful not to hinder psychoanalytic treatment.[40]

In 1959, Oraison distinguished between analysis and confession. He interpreted analysis as a medical act, while confession was a religious act. The aim of analysis was to relieve the patient of his paralyzing anxieties, not to make him immoral. Then the priest acting as a confessor gave the penitent faith, and helped him relate to God.[41]   Oraison showed a good understanding of the ways in which priests and psychoanalysts were in fact cooperating by the late 1950s and suggested that although they might perform similar-appearing functions, their roles were quite different.

Francis J. Braceland, a Catholic psychiatrist, gave further attention to the relationship between psychiatry and religion in 1959. He noted that the relationship of Catholic clergymen to psychiatrists varied greatly. In some cases priests and psychiatrists were mutually hostile, while on the other hand, there were over four hundred psychiatrists who were practicing Catholics, and many Catholic clinical psychologists.   He believed that early disagreements had been based upon the religionists' image of psychology as a man-created religion, especially one which called God-centered religion an obsessional neurosis.   Even after the theories of the neo-Freudians were accepted, Freud's religious outlook made acceptance of psychoanalysis difficult for Catholics.   In fact, Freudian psychology could be accepted, and atheistic Freudian philosophy could be rejected. Braceland said that no worthy psychiatrist would advise a patient to commit immoral sexual actions, and he emphasized that psychiatrists and priests operated within different spheres. The psychiatrist treated the emotionally ill, while the priest was capable of dealing with normal anxiety problems.[42]

Dealing with the same issue, Gustave Weigel, another theologian, suggested that the conflict between psychiatrists and theologians was the result of the psychiatrists' interest in non-materialistic subjects.   Since priests and psychiatrists were now cooperating, the greatest problem was not that psychiatrists were giving spiritual advice, but that priests were treating psychiatric problems poorly, because they lacked adequate training.[43]

A chaplain in a mental hospital could promote the integration of religion and mental health, said F. McNamee. The priest could learn from the psychiatrist about the significance of interpersonal relations, which would help man develop his relationship with God in the real world. The priest had to become a good listener, and not a judge. He had to offer acceptance and understanding through God's grace. Mental illness had to be treated by specialists, but the priest could encourage Christian love by his love of humanity.[44] McNamee's views coincided very closely with those expressed by Protestant chaplains. He believed in the effectiveness of Christian love and neo-Freudian psychology as espoused by Horney, Sullivan, and Fromm.

Religion and psychiatry could work together, asserted F. M. Limaco, if psychologists accepted religion as a scientific fact. He rejected Freudian theories, but considered that Jung's views on religion were useful. He also found the views of pastoral psychologists such as Liebman and Menninger to have positive value.

During the 1960s, Catholics became interested in the work of the pastoral psychologists of all faiths who had been writing in the post–World War II era.[45] Attempts to reconcile Freudian psychoanalysis and Thomistic philosophy also continued, with orthodox Freudianism gaining respectability, compared to the previous decades.

One of the foremost Catholic theorists who tried to reconcile psychiatry and Catholicism was John D. Higgins, a psychiatrist. He began by endorsing the Freudian psychological system as the only system which explained the cause and development of a wide range of psychological problems. Neo-Freudian revisionists had failed to develop an equally comprehensive theory, and those who accepted the neo-Freudians had failed to investigate the implications of neo-Freudian theory. Only the ego psychology of Anna Freud and Erik Erikson was compatible with the Freudian system and fit within its larger confines. Higgins said that Freud spoke of inner needs, while the neo-Freudians spoke of the social milieu.[46] An even stronger preference for Freudian over neo-Freudian ideas was expressed by Alden L. Fisher, who considered Freudian theory to be the best elucidation of man's non-spiritual mental life, and said that the Freudian unconscious did not conflict with Thomism.[47]

In the early 1960s, Catholics developed a definite concern over the effect of the non-judgmental attitude of psychiatrists upon social morality.[48]

Somewhat defensively, P. Sullivan discussed why Catholics preferred Catholic psychiatrists. Most parishioners assumed that a Catholic psychiatrist probably would have a better understanding of a patient's background than would a non-Catholic, and that he would also be less likely to give immoral advice. Sullivan postulated that the purpose of psychotherapy was to free man's behavior from irrational guilt by furnishing supportive therapy, during which the patient would learn to understand his thoughts and their origin.[49]

In 1962, Gregory Zilboorg advanced another synthesis of psychology and religion. Zilboorg contended that Freud had confused the psychic apparatus with the soul, and that most lay followers had inherited that confusion. In fact, said Zilboorg, psychology and religion were essentially separate disciplines. The Catholic sacrament of confession dealt with the conscious mind in which a sense of sin was lodged. Psychology was not equipped to deal with the soul of man, nor could it change his deep-seated ethical beliefs.

Zilboorg pointed out that Freud had dealt with *eros* or erotic love, while Christianity was concerned with a higher form of love, which was *agape* or *caritas*. *Agape* or *caritas* could only be achieved when the personality had reached a high state of organization. The philosophy of the monastic ideal had recognized the existence of genital sexuality for centuries, but suppressed it in order to further *caritas*. However, Zilboorg felt that Freud had offered valuable insights into the problem of scrupulosity. In addition, only psychology could relieve man of irrational guilt. Zilboorg concluded that rapproachement between psychology and religion was indeed possible, because psychology was now interested in morality.[50]

Thus, from 1950 to 1965 considerable progress occurred in the acceptance of psychology by Catholics. The role of psychology in the cure of mental illness was commonly acknowledged, and most Catholics now believed that neo-Freudian psychology did not conflict with Catholic philosophy. Freudian psychology still had its adherents among some intellectual Catholic psychiatrists, philosophers, and psychologists.

Questions about the morality of psychoanalysis had been mostly resolved. Psychoanalysis was moral, providing it did not employ the pansexual method of analysis, and certain aspects of the conscious mind remained closed. Thus, analysis could not involve the exploration of sexual material. In addition, all information acquired in confidence could not be discussed in psychoanalysis. Catholics were especially concerned that the secrets of the confessional be preserved at all costs. Catholic writers also attempted to resolve the problem of Freud's denial of the existence of religion, with some modicum of success.

Neo-Freudian analysts believed that religious concepts aided mental health. Catholic writers relegated Freud's anti-religious views to a minor role. They said that his atheism and materialism were nothing more than a reflection of his personal problems. Catholics uniformly rejected Freud's philosophy.

As Catholics and psychologists came into more frequent contact, and more Catholics entered the fields of psychology and psychiatry, a greater feeling of trust developed. Catholics realized that a good therapist would not recommend an immoral action. Catholics were able to distinguish moral from psychiatric problems, and the roles of the priest and the psychologist emerged as being complementary but different.

Acceptance of Freud's theories and those of the neo-Freudians came to most branches of American Judaism with comparative ease. There were many reasons for the relative absence of conflict. Jewish social service institutions had in general developed outside of the synagogue, although an occasional exception like the Free Synagogue in New York City did have a social service department. A rabbi would more typically refer people with problems to the appropriate agency, rather than give pastoral care and counseling himself. A Jewish family, seeking help for a mentally ill family member, was likely to go directly to a social service organization like the Federation of Jewish Philanthropies, and might not even discuss the problem with a rabbi. Most Jews still lived in large cities, where mental health facilities were readily available.

There was little emphasis on pastoral care in Judaism, because the rabbi traditionally spent his time praying, studying and teaching the Torah, and managing community activities such as the religious school. It was the obligation of every Jew in the community to visit and to care for the sick, and to give counsel.

In addition, traditional law mandated that a sick person himself should seek medical help. Anyone who failed to do so was considered a fool. Freud and most of the neo-Freudians were Jewish, as were most psychotherapists and many doctors in the community, and the fact that so many of the practitioners of psychology were Jewish made the acceptance of psychotherapy much easier for the Jewish community.

Rabbis began their acceptance of psychoanalysis by comparing Jewish practice with psychoanalytic theory. They were delighted to find that, in their opinion, traditional Jewish practice seemed to encourage mental health. After World War II, acceptance of psychoanalysis was evident in Reform Jewish literature, and by the 1950s, Conservative Jewish theologians were willing to accept and utilize psychoanalytic techniques.

Joshua Loth Liebman attempted the first comprehensive synthesis of Judaism with Freudian and neo-Freudian psychology in 1946. His book, entitled *Peace of Mind*,[51] was written in order to bring comfort to Jews who could not alleviate their anxieties through traditional Judaism. However, Liebman clearly stated that he was thoroughly satisfied that traditional Judaism and mysticism brought "peace of mind" to many Jews.

Liebman said that psychology and religion had similar goals, including the achievement of a good life. Prophetic religion had stressed the need for forgiveness and tolerance. Now psychology also said that man must forgive himself, and then others, before he could achieve mental health. Prophetic religion had stressed free will, and psychology only postponed the operation of free will until man's inner conflicts were resolved. Both religion and psychology aimed at making man whole.

Freud's atheism was dismissd by saying that Freud was really doing God's work. Liebman referred to the Talmud,[52] saying that a man who devoted his life to helping humanity was acceptable to God, although he might deny the existence of God. Freud, who devoted his life to curing the sick, certainly helped humanity. Liebman felt that psychology and religion had to make peace for the good of humanity. It was not necessary to accept Freud's philosophical ideas, only to utilize the understandings about the workings of the human mind which he offered.

He affirmed that moral and ethical standards had to be maintained, but the conscience, or the superego sanctions which maintained morality, had to spring from an affirmation of self-love, and not from self-hatred. Liebman sought further confirmations in the writings of Erich Fromm.[53] He concluded that a love of learning, a sense of humor, and faith in God were aids to mental health in Jewish culture.

The Jewish theologian Sol W. Ginsburg also accepted some of the basic precepts of neo-Freudian psychology. He said in 1948 that man faced three problems involving his ego, namely, the relation of man to himself, to his family, and then to the outside world. Psychology and religion should share in helping man acquire and structure a system of values which would help him achieve good interpersonal relations.[54]

Although there was little overt opposition to the acceptance of psychoanalytic techniques or theory, most Jewish theologians did not accept Freud's philosophy or his analyses of biblical history. Joshua Fishman said that there was no evidence to validate the psychological interpretation of Bible stories, and suggested that it would be more fruitful to study neurotic adults, and observe the behavior of children, than to look for abnormalities.[55] On the other hand, some Jews wanted synagogues to offer more complete mental health programs. Robert L. Katz said in 1954 that mental health programs, and educational programs which stressed the teaching of values and psychology, should be instituted in the synagogue.[56]

Jews attempted to better understand anti-Semitism by Freudian interpretation of anti-Semitic attitudes. Joseph Golnar suggested that the problem of guilt had long hindered the relationship of the Jew and the Christian. The guilt resulted from the murder of the primordial father by the horde, an experience common to all peoples. Golnar accepted Freudian social theory about the universality of the relationship of the Oedipus complex. Guilt could only be alleviated by self-acceptance, and awareness of common goals. He resolved the problems of society according to neo-Freudian theories of object relations and self-acceptance.[57]

Mortimer Ostow and Ben Ami Scharfstein said that the need to believe was as vital a necessity as eating. They did not endorse Freud's philosophical or anthropological speculations, but did accept his psychoanalytic techniques and theory. They found a link between psychiatry and religion, both in the fact that religion and psychiatry both dealt with specific human problems and experiences, such as guilt and religious and instinctual demands, and in the very nature of religion.[58]

Abraham N. Franzblau, a psychiatrist who was the chairman of the Department of Human Relations at the Hebrew Union College–Jewish Institute of Religion in New York City, held that Freud had made important contributions to the understanding of man, of which his explanation of the operation of the unconscious was most important. Franzblau said that the role of the rabbi differed significantly from that of the psychiatrist. The rabbi was supposed to believe in the efficacy of prayer, and he was sometimes expected to judge and give advice. The psychotherapist, on the other hand, was non-judgmental and often non-directive. The role of the rabbi as delineated here was quite circumscribed. He was not to do therapy, just to give counsel. According to Franzblau, the rabbi should retain his traditional role as the community wise man, but his advice should reflect an understanding of psychoanalytic concepts.[59]

Louis Linn, a psychiatrist, and Leo M. Schwarz, a rabbi, analyzed the dramatic reversal in the attitude of religious leaders to psychology. At first religious leaders had rejected psychology, because of Freud's hostile attitude towards religion. But they finally realized that traditional religious counseling was inadequate to deal with modern problems, and looked to social work and to psychiatry for new techniques which would help them counsel people.

The most important reason for the rapprochement between psychology and religion was the moral crisis of the post–World War II era, according to Linn and Schwarz. The lethal potential of atomic and hydrogen bombs, and of totalitarian societies, posed a greater moral dilemma than had hitherto been encountered. Thus, religion and psychiatry had to cooperate to help modern man curb his aggressions. They could divide the task by placing the responsibility for dealing with normal people and problems with religious leaders, while psychologists dealt with the abnormal.

Of course religion and psychiatry could not eliminate anxiety, guilt, anger, and sadness, but by working together, they could teach man how to deal with the conflicts produced by these tensions in a way which would not produce mental illness. Religion could utilize the psycho-analytical insights, while rejecting its materialistic philosophy.[60]

Simon Noveck maintained in 1956 that Judaism had a long history of acceptance of new ideas. Now psychiatric theory was offering new hypotheses about the functioning of the human mind, and demonstrating the interplay of physical and psychological factors in illness. Psychologists had also discovered that unconscious forces of repressed anger, hostility, and resentment prevented people from experiencing self-fulfillment. This was occurring at a time when religion had become increasingly insensitive to basic human needs, such as the need for love, status, security, and self-worth. Possibly pastoral counselors had an increased awareness of these problems after studying psychology.[61]

Alexander Alan Steinbach stipulated that religion and psychiatry could cooperate only within certain limits. Freud's philosophy was not compatible with religion. Religion accepted the existence of sin, and religious leaders were concerned that the acceptance of psychology might undermine morality. Religious leaders also had great difficulty in accepting the theory of infant sexuality, and especially the existence of the Oedipus and Electra complexes. Psychology and religion had different and complementary roles. The clergy still had the responsibility for solving most problems by the traditional means of faith and love, before referring the mentally ill to psychiatrists.

As Steinbach saw it, man could not discover God until he had discovered man, and religion and psychiatry could cooperate to help man achieve the good life, although there would always be disagreement about the degree of moral laxity which was permissible.[62] Certain philosophical problems remained. Steinbach met them by preferring the theories of the neo-Freudians like Horney, Fromm, and Sullivan, who emphasized the importance of good object relations, and the necessity of love of self before love of others was possible.

Abraham Franzblau also advocated cooperation between psychiatry and religion. He tried to explain Freud's anti-religious bias by assuming that some of Freud's negative religious feelings might be attributable to the deprivation he had felt when his Catholic nurse left the Freud family, and to the absence of liberal Jewish synagogues in Vienna.

Freud rejected orthodox religious groups because they depended upon creedal reaffirmation for salvation, said Franzblau. Various traditional Christian religious groups emphasized eternal damnation and forgiveness through divine grace, resurrection of the body, and the image of God as being seated upon a throne. All of these concepts were not acceptable, and would be considered regressive and neurotic by psychologists, because they emphasized the powerlessness and the worthlessness of man. Humanistic religion, which stressed growth through love and acceptance of others, was psychologically valid according to neo-Freudian psychologists.

Franzblau deduced that religion should cooperate with psychology in many areas, although psychology had to remain essentially non-judgmental, while the rabbi had many roles, and that of therapist was only one of them. He advocated the screening of all candidates for the rabbinate, to elimate those who were incapable of maintaining good object relations. Another area for cooperation was in the area of marital counseling, because ministers were more often asked for help in marital problems than were psychologists.[63] J. H. Gelberman and D. Kobak said that the emphasis on "holism" in modern Hasidism[64] was conducive to mental health.[65]

In 1958, Jacob J. Weinstein reported that the Central Conference of American Rabbis, the association of Reform rabbis, felt that no conflict existed between psychiatry and religion in the "cure of the souls." The psychiatrist was the true friend of the rabbi. Weinstein also praised the work of Jewish welfare organizations like the Jewish Family Service while noting the necessity of counseling with the rest of the family, when one member was in therapy.[66]

Many Jewish religious leaders were now stressing the importance of faith and de-emphasizing ritualism. Sandor S. Feldman declared in 1959 that the psychoanalytic meaning of Jewish religious rituals, such as circumcision, the observance of the dietary laws, and certain prayers, differed depending upon whether the observer was normal or neurotic. Reinterpretation of old rituals might cause some people to cease practicing them, but the lessening of ritual observance should not result in a decrease in faith.[67]

G. C. Anderson judged in 1963 that Jewish religious rituals were confirmed as psychologically valid.[68] The growing conviction among rabbis that Jewish religious practices were psychologically valid greatly eased the way for the absorption of psychoanalytic concepts into Judaism.

By 1965, Freudian psychology had caused a new awareness of the role of the rabbi as a pastoral counselor. Reform rabbis in particular were attracted to the neo-Freudian theories of Horney, Sullivan, and

Fromm, which stressed the importance of social and environmental factors in encouraging self-esteem and fostering good interpersonal relations. The Reform Jewish synthesis was not noticeably different from Protestant pastoral psychology in this respect.

Rabbis in general had become more aware of the existence of mental illness, and more skilled in detecting signs of illness among their congregants. However, while the impact of Freudian and neo-Freudian psychology on American-Jewish culture was extensive, there was no comparable modification in formal Judaism, in part because Jewish social service organizations existed outside the synagogue, and in part because of the traditional role and concerns of the rabbi.[69]

Theologians and Freudian Psychology

Articles criticizing and condemning Freudian psychology appeared in journals of religion long before any substantial movement for acceptance of psychoanalytic concepts developed. In these essays Protestants gave many reasons for condemning psychoanalysis. Fears were expressed that psychoanalysis would undermine social morality and supplant salvation as man's ultimate goal. Resentment of the anti-religious attitudes of most psychologists was another factor. But many critics appeared to have only the most cursory familiarity with psychoanalytic concepts.

An early article hostile to psychoanalysis was published by G. A. Coe in 1926.[1] He argued that modern psychology failed to give man enough self-recognition, and that the ideals of our society came from religion.[2] Many of these early articles seemed to Freud like one more episode in the long science versus religion controversy, with no thought about the possibilities of cooperation between the two. For example, A. E. Hayden in 1930 offered the well-worn argument that through religion a person could get a feeling of wholeness which was beyond what science could offer.[3]

K. R. Stolz wrote in 1932 that religion must remain the central experience for ministers. All changes in the structure of the personality had to be rooted in religion, because religion was concerned with the ultimate reality.[4] H. C. Link expressed the same point of view in 1936, declaring that psychological adjustments had to be made through religion.[5] In 1927 H. N. Wieman affirmed that salvation was the way to cure human problems.[6] A. J. Jorden was concerned about the primacy of religion in 1927. He charged that psychology was making its own religion; religion, therefore, had to make its own psychology. Warning that psychologists should not involve themselves in theology which was the exclusive province of religionists, he called conscience an "innate force" which guaranteed that man would always aspire towards the divine.[7] P. B. Herring said that the study of the Gospels was the Christian method of healing all complexes.[8]

Although religious authorities rejected the new psychologies, by the 1930s they were beginning to use the new psychoanalytic vocabulary,

including words such as complexes, ego, id, and superego. Psychoanalytic terminology became a part of popular American culture before
the theory itself.

In 1947 Paul E. Johnson, who was later to advocate the use of
psychoanalytic concepts by Christian counselors, still relied upon
traditional methods of relieving suffering. He said that feelings of guilt
could be assuaged by forgiveness, and that sorrow could be overcome
through confession. However, the attainment of mental health was an
important goal which led to feelings of increased personal worth and the
ultimate triumph of good over evil. He urged that people guide the
young into paths of worship and a disciplined way of life.[9]

The journals of the more theologically conservative Protestant
denominations remained almost unanimous in their opposition to the
incursion of psychoanalytic concepts. For instance, E. Steinhal wrote in
the *Lutheran Quarterly* that man could know himself through God, and
therefore he did not need the ministrations of psychoanalysts.[10]

The journals of psychology and religion favorable to Freud, such as
the *Journal of Pastoral Care* and *Pastoral Psychology,* printed some
articles which cautioned against the adoption of psychoanalytic concepts
by religionists. The editors of *Pastoral Psychology* said that the pastor
could never be objective when counseling. He would always be trying to
bring man closer to God by utilizing the techniques of confession,
repentance, forgiveness, faith and obedience. Referral to psychoanalysts
represented interruptions in pastoral care.[11] Doris Mode in 1950
preferred God-centered over client-centered therapy. She insisted that
neurotic patients were self-centered already and did not need a therapy
which increased their concentration on themselves. Mode preferred
Christian God-centered therapy based upon surrender to God and
utilizing the technique of confession and salvation. She said that free
will was possible only under conditions of surrender to God.[12]

Anton Boisen who worked hard to establish clinical training
programs for ministers expressed doubts about the value of specialized
training and techniques. He said that "interpersonal relationships of
understanding and friendship" were the most important aids in a
counseling situation. Boisen felt that some forms of mental illness,
especially those where feelings of anxiety and of sinfulness were present,
were actually manifestions of health. The real evils were not sin but
human isolation and estrangement from mankind which developed when
instinctual demands could not be controlled or acknowledged. Love,
according to Boisen, was the paramount human need.[13] Although Boisen
de-emphasized specialized techniques and training, the influence of the
neo-Freudians was clear in his discussion of the nature and cure of neuroses.

David E. Roberts in 1952 reminded readers that only Christianity offered integration on the highest level which could end man's isolation. Psychotherapy by itself left man "autonomous."[14] He emphasized that counseling should take place in a clearly Christian context with the goal of religious conversion or acceptance of God clearly in view at all times. Christian therapy, as he envisioned it, could not be non-directive or client-centered.

In 1952 Samuel Miller wrote that not everyone ought to be socially and personally adjusted. He noted that St. Francis of Assisi, William Wilberforce, and Thomas Paine had not been well adjusted and yet had performed many good deeds.[15] Also, Joachim Scharfenberg said that modern psychology could not develop a psychology of man nor could it prepare man for the second coming of Christ.[16] W. Earl Biddle argued in 1952 that a truly scientific depth psychology did conflict with the theory of free will. He found the psychoanalytic explanation of interpersonal relations unsatisfactory because it limited the operation of the mind. Union with God was the ultimate goal of all interpersonal relationships. It was Biddle's impression that Freud regarded the individual as oppressed by the morality and standards established by the leaders of the group in order to preserve their power.[17]

Gradually articles became increasingly selective and sophisticated in their criticism of the influence of psychology on religion. By the 1950s many writers displayed a mastery of psychoanalytic terms and concepts, and tended to object only to some particular aspect of pastoral psychology. But, there remained an ever present and overriding concern for retaining the primacy of Christianity in pastoral counseling and insuring that attainment of mental health would lead man to behave according to Christian ideals. An instance of that concern was the comment of George O. Evenson in 1953 that although integration of the personality was a "laudable" goal, unless the personality was integrated in Jesus Christ, the minister was betraying his trust.[18]

Newer sophistication was demonstrated in Orville S. Walters' 1953 article praising Rogerian client-centered therapy because its techniques discouraged a minister from being too talkative. Nevertheless Walters criticized Rogerian therapy for lacking a fixed morality and for containing naturalistic and humanistic elements which made its therapy irreconcilable with Christian doctrine.[19]   In 1954 A. T. Molligen announced that analysts who considered God a delusion did not really understand what delusions were. Analysts should study the religious and the philosophical implications of finitude and the purpose of existence.[20] G. C. Anderson agreed that psychiatrists should be competent to deal with moral problems.[21]

In spite of growing sophistication, some writers remained cautious about Freud as the decade advanced. Milton Rosenberg in 1957 described the outlook of Norman Vincent Peale and Joshua Loth Liebman who, Rosenberg said, considered psychic cleanliness as being next to godliness. Rosenberg did not think that psychotherapy would insure salvation and at the same time improve an individual's personality.[22] Gibson Winter said that the newly trained pastoral psychologists were so uncertain of their proper role that many were leaving the ministry. Winter suggested that pastoral visits to alcoholics, the mentally ill, and the sick could be performed by laymen. The clergyman should then confine himself to helping people grow in the fellowship of the Gospels and of the sacraments.[23]

Russell B. Blelzer in 1957 asserted that a minister could not be an ecclesiastical psychiatrist. He could not receive negative transference feelings from counselees and still act as a group leader and as a preacher. Blelzer felt that the minister should not have a regular schedule of counseling duties. Any person who required counseling on a regular basis should be referred to a social service agency.[24]

C. Bergendoff in 1958 did not deny the importance of Freudian theories, but stressed that psychology belonged to the material world, which was not as important as the preservation of the concept of the trinity or the recognition of God's power.[25] David Elton Trueblood disagreed with Freud's statement that religion was infantile wish-fulfillment.[26] A. W. Clark said in 1963 that complete faith in God was necessary, with neither conventional faith nor psychiatry a sufficient substitute, although a scientific education was important.[27]

Finally, Donald A. Krill claimed in 1965 that neuroses and psychoses were caused by a person behaving in a manner which violated his conscience. He considered that all guilt was real, because emotional problems resulted from misdeeds during which the id dominated the ego and the superego. Krill thought that the proper treatment of misdeeds was confession and changed behavior. He said that psychoanalysis resulted in self-pity on the part of the patient.[28]

People continued to be concerned about the morality of psychoanalysis; they expressed this anxiety in the lay journals of opinion during the 1960s. In 1960 O. S. Walters felt sure that psychiatry could not be ethically neutral. The psychiatrist should have some knowledge of Christianity.[29]

That same year, P. Landon stated that morality and Christianity were more important than Freudian psychology.[30] O. S. Walters reaffirmed that there was room for cooperation between psychology and religion, but there were also problems because psychology did not unquestioningly accept the moral precepts of religion. The greatest potential for conflict existed when the patient's neuroses were linked to religion, because psychologists had difficulty distinguishing between normal and abnormal religiosity.[31] W. Harden added that Freud had failed to find the cure for man's suffering, with special reference to O. H. Mowrer's theory that in a neurosis the superego suppressed guilt which was the accepted cause of neurosis. It was necessary to acknowledge guilt and receive forgiveness in order to attain salvation.[32]

Pre–World War II critiques of Freudian psychology indicate that the major Catholic concern was over the conflict between the permissive attitudes towards morality suggested by Freudian theory and the moral teachings of the Church. Another conflict involved Freud's antireligious attitudes and Catholic doctrine. Often Catholic writers seemed not to have grasped the significance of Freudian technique and theory, for they dwelt heavily upon his philosophy, which was more shocking to a Catholic and easier to understand than his psychoanalytic theories or techniques.

M. Stendin in 1930 labeled experimental psychology cold and inhuman.[33] C. H. Williamson in 1932 thought that Freudian psychology was a mere fad. He placed more emphasis on Freudian philosophy and psychology than on Freudian techniques.[34] Also in 1932, W. H. Sheldon reaffirmed the Catholic doctrine of the supremacy of the rational mind. He said that the mind acted upon the body; the body did not act upon the mind as Freud stated in his theory of unconscious motivation.[35] In 1937 W. P. Commins granted that psychology might have some value, but lamented that it lacked a general philosophy.[36] O'Brien compared the psychoanalytic method with the sacrament of confession and concluded that confession offered catharsis and was superior to psychoanalysis because it preserved anonymity.[37] Some Catholic writers did not think that psychoanalysis was effective in the treatment of mental illness. W. J. Gerry said that a spanking was more useful than psychoanalysis. He objected to the pansexuality and materialism of Freudian psychology, which he felt was a threat to morality and to man's free will.[38]

Rudolf Allers in 1939 briefly discussed the process of psychoanalysis and Freudian philosophy. He concluded that there was no satisfactory psychoanalytic treatment for Catholics because no method of psychoanalysis dealt with the problem of morality.[39] J. W. Stafford noted that outside of Catholic philisophical circles the doctrine of free will was rejected, although man had to have free will if he was rational.[40] M. Kant observed in 1943 that Freud had overlooked the aspect of man which made him different from other animals, namely, his immortal soul. Kant did not believe that man's motivating force was his libido.[41]

At the beginning of the postwar era, many Catholics still thought that the Church could cure mental illness.[42] K. Novis found many things to criticize in Freudian psychology. It destroyed man's sense of responsibility while it increased his egotism. Psychology offered a coarse, sexually oriented explanation of all problems and decreased man's spirituality. Novis concluded that a person could find better solutions to his problems within his family.[43] Novis did not seem to understand the nature of mental illness.

Agnostic elements in Jungian psychology made it unacceptable to Catholics, said Karl Stern.[44] In 1950, J. B. Scheeva suggested that the attitude of Catholics towards pychoanalysis should be one of watchful waiting. He thought that man could not be dealt with as an animal, ignoring his spiritual qualities, and felt that the psychological goal of social adjustment differed from the Christian goal of salvation. Scheeva also considered that confession was preferable to analysis.[45]

The genuine conflicts between Catholic teaching and Freudian psychology were beginning to emerge. They included the debate over the efficacy of confession as an alternative to psychoanalysis, and the supremacy of the rational mind over the unconscious irrational mind. Catholics were also concerned about the problems involved in the maintenance of absolute moral standards as the patients progressed towards a better social adjustment. Freud's denial of the existence of God and of man's soul troubled them greatly.

A. Stander objected to psychoanalysis because it was based upon man's irrationality; he urged Catholics to develop a rational Christian psychology.[46] Some Catholics still failed to distinguish between normal and neurotic guilt. They said that the guilt feelings of the individual were useful in maintaining social morality.[47] A. Keenan thought that neuroses were part of Christian suffering, and psychoanalysis was immoral.[48] Similar in view was D. Dohen's idea that neuroses could be cured through baptism and rebirth; thus, neuroses could be beneficial.[49]

In 1952, Catholic periodicals reported on the condemnation by Pope Pius XII of Freudian psychology.[50] G. F. George noted that the Pope opposed the pansexual method of psychoanalysis, and the analysis of dreams and free association.[51] Catholic moral teachings could not be replaced by psychology.[52] This was followed by a sharp increase in hostile Catholic press opinions.

In 1956, J. B. McAllister, a cleric, said that almost all aspects of psychoanalysis were indebted to Freudian theory and had to be rejected. He considered that Freudian psychoanalysis undermined morality and society. If psychoanalysis were accepted he did not know how individual lives were to be reconstructed. McAllister said that real guilt existed and that misdeeds had to be expiated. He was opposed to the idea of unconscious motivation carried to the degree that man stopped relying upon the sacraments of the Church for the remission of sins. He was afraid that psychoanalysis would replace confession and repentance as the method of remitting sins.[53]

J. M. Martin explained the special role of the Catholic psychiatrist. He was to serve mankind by treating the whole man and must do nothing to diminish free will or to deny the objective nature of sin. The Catholic psychiatrist should explore hagiography to show how the saints had struggled against obsessional neuroses. They should also study incidences of stigmata and help screen candidates for religious life and counsel "troubled" sisters in religious life.[54]

R. B. Nording said that the denial of man's rationality was the biggest stumbling block in the way of reconciling psychology and religion. Man's rationality was one of the most important concepts in Christianity. Psychoanalysts would have to admit that man was pre-eminently rational and that rationality was desirable before psycho-analysis and Christianity could ever work together.[55] R. A. De Nardo said in 1958 that psychoanalysis prevented man from yearning for God and for salvation.[56]

In 1958, Pope Pius XII issued a more sweeping condemnation of Freudian psychology, but with a postscript that, within the limits of Catholic moral teaching, other methods of psychoanalysis were acceptable to Catholics.[57] M. E. Steck interpreted the Pope's condemnation as the result of Freud's emphasis on sexual origin of neuroses, the sexual interpretation of dreams, and investigation of sexual thought in free association. He repeated the advice of John Ford to patients undergoing psychoanalysis. They were not to accept immoral advice. They were to be aware of problems which might result from the formation of transference or countertransference neuroses, and they might not acquiesce to immoral fantasies which might be released by free association.[58]

Since few Catholic writers did more than grudgingly acknowledge the usefulness of psychology in treating mental illness, often acceptance and rejection existed on a continuum rather than in direct contrast. Most Catholic writers who went on rejecting psychoanalysis in the 1950s and 1960s did so because they feared that psychoanalytic theory would undermine morality and the teachings of the Church. They thought that psychoanalysis concentrated on what they considered to be man's more animalistic aspect while it de-emphasized his spirituality. Other writers still seemed to have a poor idea of the nature and symptoms of mental illness.

There was almost no opposition by Jewish theologians to the acceptance of psychoanalytic concepts. Those who were less interested in psychology continued studying the traditional religious books. Their inattention, combined with the existence of Jewish social service organizations outside of the synagogue and the high respect in which doctors and medical knowledge were held in the Jewish community, resulted in very little opposition to the assimilation of psychological concepts into Jewish thought and life.

Effect of Psychological Concepts on Theology

The influence of neo-Freudian and Freudian psychology upon religion can be seen clearly and strongly in the discussion of such traditional concerns as anxiety and notions of sexuality. These and other aspects of human behavior were dealt with in terms of an individual's need for good interpersonal relations, rather than their value to society.

The battle for acceptance of Freudian and neo-Freudian psychology was successfully fought in the 1950s; the leaders of the battle had experienced World War II and the Great Depression. Although theologians tended to react slowly to contemporary culture, they were of the society and could not help but be influenced by the prevailing modes of thought and attempts to make all aspects of man's life relevant to his experience. Hence, all aspects of the culture tended to reflect the changes which rapidly occurred in postwar society.

Theologians sought to reconcile psychology and religion by recognizing the function which psychologists seemed to be able to perform best — the cure of the mentally ill — and by reviewing traditional religious concepts and practices to insure that they were psychologically valid. They did not seek to radically revise Christianity or Judiasm, but rather to enrich and to improve religion. When change did occur, it was naturally concentrated in those areas which were of special concern in the postwar era.

Theologians paid the greatest attention to problems of anxiety and guilt. Modern man, often depicted by neo-Freudian psychologists as being alienated from himself, his fellow man, his environment and ultimately from his god, was a familiar figure in the post–World War II United States. Americans had sustained many types of severe anxiety in the middle twentieth century, with one type following another in too rapid succession for many people to fully accustom themselves to one set of problems before they had to confront an entirely new type of anxiety-producing situation. During the 1930s, economic problems were the primary anxiety-provoking experience. The real recovery from the economic woes of the depression occurred during World War II, which caused another and different set of anxieties, including battlefield anxieties and anxieties caused by the disruption of families through the induction of men into the armed forces, the entrance of women into the labor force, and the resettlement of families into areas where defense industries offered employment.   In addition to the usual difficulties in readjusting to life in peacetime, Americans had to cope with horrors which had never before been envisioned, including the Holocaust and the destructive potentials of nuclear warfare.

In the postwar era the question of guilt had to be re-examined. Soldiers returned from the war feeling guilt over wartime acts. Men had participated in mass murder on a scale that was previously unimaginable, and yet experienced little or no guilt. Theologians felt that the existence of guilt, whether or not it was sensed by the individual, had to be examined. The sinner was now seen as a sick rather than evil individual. The greater a person's psychological health, the more readily he could avoid sin and obey God's commandments in a spirit of love and of acceptance, and the greater the ease with which he could withstand the normal burdens of life.   Therefore, the focus of religion shifted from condemning the sinner to helping him through the experience of love *(agape)* to attain sufficient feelings of relatedness and personal integration so that he could acknowledge his sins and accept God's forgiveness, and salvation.

Theologians also examined the problems of mysticism, worship, and conversion in the light of neo-Freudian psychology, but there was relatively little interest in the practices of mysticism or in liturgical changes at this time. Conversion experiences were examined in terms of their effect upon the psychological health and organization of the individual.

Originally, Freud's statements about the role of sexual drive in man were emphasized in order to frighten people away from a careful examination of his theories, but as the twentieth century wore on, it was clear that the heyday of Victorian sexual morality was passing. Freud's ideas about the importance of a healthy sexuality as part of the full development of the individual were used to rationalize and explain pervasive changes in attitudes towards sex. Sexual morality was changing because of new methods of contraception which lessened fear of pregnancy as the reason for sexual abstinence, the breakup of the family as an economic and social unit, and the increasing employment of women outside of the home. Therefore, theologians reviewed traditional religious attitudes towards sexuality in terms of what was beneficial to the society as well as to the individual, and tried to find a middle ground which would allow for psychologically sound sexual expression within the family-oriented structure of society. Most of the battle for liberalization of sexual morals was fought elsewhere than in the journals and books of pastoral psychology and theology. The response of the theologians was mostly an attempt to come to terms with an existing condition which varied from traditional, religiously oriented practice.

Anxiety

The influence of psychology on the theory of anxiety was greatest for Protestant theologians, who were especially aware of the crippling effects of anxiety on every aspect of human life in the post–World War II era. Anxiety in everyday life, in man's relationship with God, and as a form of mental illness concerned them. Difficulty arose in differentiating ontological or existential anxiety from neurotic anxiety as defined by non-religious psychologists.

Protestant theologians accepted Freudian theory about the dynamic nature of anxiety as an internalized threat to the individual's existence, and neo-Freudian theory about the social causes of anxiety as the result of deficient self-esteem and poor object relations. Usually, they felt that the sacraments and the fellowship offered by religion could help alleviate non-neurotic and finitude anxiety. Neurotic anxiety was a mental health problem which involved the pastor to the extent that his feeling of competence as a pastoral counselor permitted.

On the other hand, existential psychologists believed that existential anxiety was one of man's greatest problems. It could be alleviated only by faith in God, acceptance of others, and self-acceptance. Ultimately, this process would lead to self-realization.

Early discussions were rather elementary. Psychologist R. R. Willoughby wrote in 1935 that magic and similar practices were defenses to neutralize anxiety. He added that different cultures generated different amounts of anxiety.[1] A traditional Christian statement on the cure for anxiety was offered in 1948, when Roger B. Nichols postulated that "reconciliation, conversion, and salvation" were the cure for anxiety.[2]

The problem of anxiety was of great concern to existential psychologists, because they were not only concerned with normal and neurotic anxiety, but also with existential anxiety. Rollo May differentiated between "creative" and neurotic anxiety. He suggested that most religious writers focused upon "creative" anxiety, which was the anxiety man felt about the reason for, and the nature of human existence. Religious writers hoped that "creative" anxiety would cause man to seek God and find alleviation through faith.

May felt that real or existential (creative) anxiety could be used by sick people to hide neurotic anxiety from themselves. Normal anxiety was part of all human existence. May conceded that religious beliefs and practices might be used to overcome normal or neurotic anxiety. Religion was a neurotic method of allaying the basic anxiety which resulted from man's isolation, but used creatively, religion could help man deal with the human condition. May credited Freud and Niebuhr with saying that all creative endeavor was stimulated by anxiety. May said that psychiatrists had not explored ontological anxiety, which was discussed by Tillich.[3]

Anxiety as defined by May was a threat to one's self, one's existence, or one's values. He noted Pfister's work on fear and religion.[4] May summarized Freud's views on anxiety as repressed libido which was transformed and then expressed indirectly as anxiety. Later, when the ego sensed danger in the outer world, it used anxiety as a means of repression. He then offered a neo-Freudian definition: anxiety developed when the possibility of rejection in interpersonal relationships existed. The degree of anxiety was in proportion to the importance of the relationship to the people being rejected. Anxiety occurred when a basic threat to the individual arose; it reflected a gap between expectation and reality, which had originally developed in the relationship between the parent and the child, and represented a contradiction between expectations and reality.[5]

Anton Boisen, the father of the clinical training movement, said that anxiety was a protective device against personal failure, not the core of neurotic personality structures, as depicted by certain modern psychiatrists. Boisen charged that modern psychiatrists were not sufficiently aware of the cultural factors in anxiety. He believed that anxiety could motivate a change in personality structure, which would precipitate a conversion experience, which was the ultimate aim of pastoral counseling.[6]

Another psychiatrist, Earl Bond, discussed anxiety in 1951. Some anxiety was good for man, he thought, but neurotic anxiety prevented man from knowing peace. Anxiety could be a free-floating feeling of mental uneasiness, which could be attached to phobias. Relief from anxiety could be found by converting the anxiety into physical symptoms.[7]

The following year Samuel H. Miller declared that mental health could not be obtained simply by releasing repressions. Basic anxiety preceded and created repression. Therefore, it was the basic anxiety which needed treatment, and the best treatment of anxiety was the creation of a deep sense of security and belongingness, accompanied by sense of reality. A person who was not secure in his relationship with others, and with his environment, could not tolerate the uncertainties which accompanied freedom of thought and action, and would have to regress to a more repressive pattern.[8]

Isidor Thorner emphasized the beneficial effect of anxiety in 1953. He felt that the anxiety in ascetic Protestant denominations, in combination with good social relations, reduced the incidence of neurosis in those groups.[9]

The interpretation by Fred Berthold of the theological meaning of anxiety as found in the writings of St. Theresa of Avila was similar. Berthold agreed that anxiety was polar. It could either be creative or destructive, and it underlaid anxiety about the proper fulfillment of life. Modern existential psychologists later termed that kind of anguish existential anxiety. Berthold noted that anxiety could also be a reaction to a loved one who was endangered. Another type of anxiety was anxiety about death and the perfection of life. Berthold did not believe that anxiety indicated estrangement from God. He thought that it signified a disturbed, but unbroken and basically healthy relationship between God and man.[10]

Wayne E. Oates discussed anxiety in *Anxiety in the Christian Experience*[11] in 1955. He listed various types of anxiety including economic anxiety, which could be beneficial because they clarified personal relationships, although an excess of economic anxiety could be devastating. He noted that wealth was seen as a sign of God's favor in the Old Testament, and poverty was seen as evidence of hidden sin. In the New Testament, man tried to win salvation and security through work.

Another type of anxiety was finitude anxiety, or the fear of death. In a neurotic individual, finitude anxiety could result in insanity or suicide. In a healthy person, it stimulated the search for God and for faith.

Grief resulting from the death of a loved one was yet another type of anxiety. Believing that grief anxiety was really suppressed hostility, reconciliation through forgiveness was the method for overcoming grief. Through reconciliation and forgiveness, it was possible to overcome sin, and sin was the greatest cause of disruption in human relationships. Sin led to isolation, which was the greatest social evil. He also wrote of legalistic anxiety, which occurred when the law stood in the way of redemption.

Oates argued that people who failed to show anxiety in the face of sin demonstrated a lack of relatedness to trusted people whose approval mattered to the individual. Amoral people reflected an amoral upbringing. It was the job of the pastor to bring Christian love to the isolated individual, and to awaken his moral sense. His last type, anxiety of the holy dread, he described as the awe that a high-minded person felt in the presence of God.

Thus, Oates distinguished many types of normal anxiety which were a part of daily living, apart from neurotic and finitude anxiety. He realized that excessive anxiety of any variety could be devastating to the entire personality, and that anxiety could camouflage hostility after a bereavement, or indicate the presence of sin. He accepted the neo-Freudian formulation of sin; the sinner was a sick person, and the existence of sin indicated a lack of relatedness to other people.

The Freudian-oriented Calvin S. Hall explained Freud's definition of anxiety in 1955. He said that anxiety existed in normal persons, and played a central role in Freud's theory of neuroses and psychoses, and in the treatment of mental illness. Anxiety was fear which was directed toward an internal object. Hall also differentiated between real and neurotic anxiety.[12] In an environmentally focused article, John Sutherland Bonnell noted that the postwar era was an age of anxiety. He attributed pervasive anxiety to the threat of war, the fear of the recurrence of the Great Depression, and anxiety which was derived from guilt. Only religious faith could provide relief from anxiety.[13]

One of the critics best known to the general public was Karl Menninger, who joined the discussion of anxiety in 1963. To Menninger anxiety was a danger signal, which, if not heard because it was repressed, could result in phobias, severe neuroses, or hysteria. He listed three types of anxiety, which he called objective (real) anxiety, neurotic anxiety, and moral anxiety. Menninger felt that earlier theories of neurotic anxiety had considered it only frustrated excitation.

He then criticized current theological theories of anxiety. In his judgment, Reinhold Niebuhr thought that anxiety was derived from sin, and that man was both free, or the possessor of free will, and finite. Paul Tillich considered that anxiety was existential, and that neurotic, or pathological, anxiety was warped existential anxiety. The root of man's anxiety, according to Tillich, was in man's existential condition, his concern about his finitude, and the nature of human existence.[14]

Religiously speaking, Albert Outler was more conventional in calling anxiety both neurotic and ontological at the same time. Anxiety was neurotic to the extent that it misconstrued "man's groundlessness," which was anxiety about his descent into hell. Outler thought that only through faith in God could man find the "ground" to end the anxiety.[15]

In an important 1964 essay, Randolf Miller surveyed the ways in which the church could reduce anxiety. He said that the acceptance offered by the church through fellowship and the sacraments was always an antidote to anxiety. The process began with the sacrament of infant baptism, which lessened maternal anxiety. Then he added that the development of anxiety led to undesirable compromises, such as attempts to escape to "second best" solutions, and fantasy, or lapsing into apathy.

Miller next considered the causes of anxiety throughout the

different stages in the child's development. He was particularly influenced by Sullivan's theories. Thus he asserted that parental anxiety about their children's behavior and development could be diminished by counseling; useful material was available which instructed parents on the way to introduce children to religion, and to prepare them for the experience of Sunday school without producing anxiety in the children. Learning to get along with their peers reduced anxiety in children, said Miller, while the strengthening of peer relationships diminished the previously absolute dependence of the children on the parents, though it somewhat reduced the parents' stature in the children's eyes. As the child entered adolescence, the sexual instincts became the chief source of anxiety. At this time the fellowship of the church could help; the adolescent integrated himself into his family and community, and in his relationship with God.[16] Miller thought that Sullivan's view of anxiety was optimistic here, but there was always hope that anxiety could be diminished.

Miller's understanding of the stages of normal anxiety was quite sophisticated and demonstrated familiarity with the theories of the neo-Freudians.

In his opinion, the resolution of ontological, or existential, anxiety was only a small part of the role that the church and the pastor should play in the lessening of anxiety. He believed that normal anxiety presented a real problem to the average individual. The causes of anxiety changed as the individual developed; there were various ways of combating anxiety, including fellowship, counseling, and education.

The influence of psychology on Catholic thought, as it related to the problem of anxiety, lay in the recognition of neurotic anxiety as a psychiatric rather than a moral problem. Odenwald and VanderVeldt recognized that there was a difference between neurotic and normal anxiety. Normal anxiety could be alleviated by the sacraments of the Church, including confession, penance, and forgiveness. Neurotic anxiety was a psychiatric problem, and would not be alleviated by the sacraments. If an anxiety neurosis was caused by frustrated sexual urges, then the patient should be so informed, in order that he might confront his problem realistically. Sexual abstinence might cause anxiety neurosis, when the abstinence was motivated by the fear of marriage and of having children, or by scrupulosity.[17]

The neurotic bore less moral responsibility for sins committed in a state of anxiety. There was some sentiment among Catholic writers that anxiety was beneficial, to the extent that it stopped people from violating the moral teachings of the Church.

Jewish theologians were particularly concerned about anxiety, because many Jews suffered from anxiety neuroses. Jewish writers tried to explain the high incidence of neuroses and psychosomatic illnesses among Jews in terms of special environmental pressures on them. Jewish theologians also differentiated between real and neurotic anxiety. They said that religious faith in God, in eternal life, and in the goodness of terrestrial life could alleviate normal anxiety, but neurotic anxiety was a psychiatric problem. In general, Jewish writers accepted the neo-Freudian theories of Horney, Fromm, and Sullivan about the social causes of neuroses. They urged the maintenance of democracy, and self-acceptance, and the acceptance of others as the best cures and pre-ventatives of anxiety neuroses.

Joshua Loth Liebman differentiated between normal and abnormal fear, or anxiety. In his early synthesis of religion and psychiatry, he said that it was necessary to accept help from others, and to accept one's own limitations in order to master fear,[18] but it was also necessary to stop worshipping success. Every man had to set his own goals by determining what was necessary for his family. Religious faith in God and in an afterlife also eased anxieties. Liebman accepted neo-Freudian theories about the importance of self-acceptance and interpersonal relations.

Some Jews thought that neuroses, particularly anxiety neuroses, and anxiety related psychosomatic ailments were more prevalent among Jews than among the general populaton. Henry Raphael Gold[19] attributed the higher incidence of neuroses and psychosomatic ailments to twenty centuries of intermittent persecution, which he said mobilized inner anxieties. He said that some Jews dealt with their anxieties by identifying with the dominant culture to the extent of denying their Jewish culture. Such Jews distorted their spiritual life and developed feelings of inferiority, which could lead to self-hatred and self-destruction through psychosomatic illness.

Jews often experienced anxiety when they had to adapt to new cultures quickly. One manifestation of anxiety was the feelings of inferiority which drove many Jews to seek success compulsively, in order to prove themselves worthy of acceptance. The compulsive drive for success caused many Jews to worship material success, and denigrate spiritual values.[20]

Henry Enoch Kagan thought that the main source of anxiety was man's need to be needed, and the fear that he would not be needed. He accepted Fromm's theories about the social causes of neuroses, and those of Horney and Sullivan about the need of self-acceptance and good interpersonal relations as the cure for anxiety. Political dictatorships, he suggested, arose because people sought to alleviate their anxieties by regressing to a childlike dependent relationship with a father figure.

Anxiety could cause hysterical symptoms and aimless motivation in an individual. Kagan believed that religion could alleviate anxiety. In addition, the individual could develop a feeling of belonging, and the fellowship which would help him conquer anxiety. Kagan said that Judaism stressed the supreme importance of each individual.[21]

Thus, theologians were concerned about types of normal, neurotic, and ontological anxiety, because they felt that modern man was especially prey to these anxieties. The influence of psychology can be seen in their skill in differentiating normal from neurotic anxiety, and in their realization that the neurotic sufferer from anxiety needed psychotherapy in addition to pastoral care. Theologians were delighted that the sacraments of the church and the prayers of atonement in Judiasm had the effect of alleviating anxiety and guilt in normal people, as did the fellowship offered by all religious groups. Psychologists and theologians continued to uphold differing views about the nature of ontological or finitude anxiety.

Guilt

Psychological theories about the effectiveness of guilt, as opposed to love, as a motivating force in human behavior caused theologians to re-examine theories about the nature of guilt.

Protestant theologians continued to believe that guilt really did exist, but they changed their views about the absence of guilt. Traditionally, Protestant theologians had accepted the existence of guilt as evidence of unconfessed and unrepented sins. A clear conscience was taken to be the sign of a righteous person. Those who seemed to be unduly burdened by guilt, without visible reason, were considered very sensitive in matters pertaining to guilt. Neurotic guilt had to be overcome before God's forgiveness could be accepted. Theologians were also interested in the roots of guilt in the conscious and the unconscious mind, and in the proper identification of sins, the commission of which precipitated the guilt. The acceptance of neo-Freudian theories of interpersonal relations caused theologians to insist that, in order to repent one's sins fully and to receive God's forgiveness, one had to have good object relations.

The earliest impact of Freudian psychology on Protestant thought about guilt was the differentiation between real and neurotic guilt. This conception caused theologians to distinguish between real guilt, which was caused by the commission of sin, and false or neurotic guilt, which was guilt over imaginary sins, sometimes called scrupulosity. Scrupulosity could not be dealt with effectively by the traditional sacramental methods of confession, forgiveness and repentance. It had neurotic roots in the person's unconscious mind, and could only be alleviated through psychotherapy.

Protestant pastoral psychologists in the post–World War II era emphasized that guilt was real, and indicative of the presence of sin. A person who did not feel guilt was not necessarily virtuous. He probably was alienated from himself and from his environment, and was unable to relate to either himself or to his environment sufficiently to develop feelings of guilt. On the other hand, the person who was overwhelmed by guilt was probably suffering from neurotic guilt, and needed psychotherapeutic help, just as the amoral person did. The normal virtuous person experienced some guilt feelings, which could be alleviated by participating in the sacraments and the fellowship of the church.

In 1950, John Sutherland Bonnell, a New York City minister, wrote that irrational guilt was the province of psychiatrists. Divine prayer and forgiveness through confession should alleviate the guilt which resulted from moral transgression.[22] A neurotic person might have moral lapses which he could not control. His problems were in the domain of the psychiatrist, and his lapses could be excused because of his lack of control. Bonnell did not believe that a person possessed complete free will.[23]

Rollo May discussed speculation over the causes of guilt from Victorian times to the post–World War II era, and the way in which problems of guilt had changed to problems of self-alienation. May thought that guilt in Victorian times arose when the sexual instincts came into conflict with Victorian morality. Then the dominant neurotic guilt feelings caused by sexual repression or feelings of inadequacy and inferiority caused by the inability to assume the mature role demanded by society. By the 1930s, a dependent, anxious and guilt-ridden type, whose outward symptoms were vocational failure and rebelliousness towards society, was a common figure. Instead of self-affirmation as his goal, this neurotic individual lived in order to please others, and experienced guilt because of his inability to fulfill societal or parental expectations. In the post–World War II era, problems of guilt were overshadowed by character disorders resulting from self-alienation. The problem of alleviating guilt became part of the larger problem of enabling an individual to accept his entire self and others.[24]

Other Protestant-oriented critics gave attention to other aspects of the guilt question. J. Hoffman, in 1952, distinguished between neurotic and real guilt. He said that the resolution of unconscious guilt feelings, which were a type of neurotic guilt, was the job of the psychiatrist.[25] In

1963, Erich Lindeman noted that there was a relationship on the part of the bereaved between grief and guilt. He said that morbid guilt feelings could be counteracted by divine grace, although real grief work had to be done to emancipate the mourner from the deceased.[26]

Adolf Koberle was particularly interested in the religious dimensions of guilt. He asserted that the pastor had a special role in the alleviation of guilt, which was the granting of absolution, and that absolution went beyond the relief that psychotherapy could offer. Koberle then turned to the views of Jung and Freud on guilt. As he saw it, Freud had attributed guilt to conflicts arising from the sexual instincts. On the other hand, Jung had placed guilt in the depth of the soul in the "shadow." Koberle suggested that man must learn to accept the fourth dark force which existed in addition to the trinity, and make productive use of it. This would entail acceptance of the complexity of guilt.[27]

Le Roy Alden gave his attention to the roots of guilt. He noted that Freud had traced guilt back into the patient's history, and that Augustine had said that all human experience was cumulative. Therefore, it was necessary to explore the past in order to find the true sources of guilt. Without discovering the origin, it was impossible to resolve guilt properly, or to prevent its recurrence. Alden argued that it was possible to interpose "egocentric desire" to deny the true source of guilt, and to attribute one's guilt to a more favorable source. Alden added that masochistic individuals could seek a "guilt-ridden" life style to satisfy the demands of an involuted ego. In such a case, he said, the aggressive instincts, which were part of the death instinct, were turned inward by the superego. A guilt-ridden person might suffer guilt feelings before every act, but that kind of guilt was neurotic, not moral or religious guilt, and would have to be treated as a psychological problem. Real guilt could be fully faced only in an atmosphere of forgiveness.[28]

Leon M. Salzman insisted that neo-Freudians distinguished between true and false guilt. True guilt existed on a conscious level. It developed when an individual took responsibility for his actions.[29]

Catholic theologians never doubted the reality of guilt. However, they became increasingly willing and able to distinguish between real and neurotic guilt, and to realize that the former was a religious problem, while the latter was a psychiatric problem.

Odenwald and VanderVeldt recognized both neurotic and rational guilt. A rational person felt real guilt after sinning. Some sinners felt compunction and remorse, and feared divine punishment after sinning. However, this sense of guilt was ended by confession, and the reception of God's forgiveness.

But neurotic guilt was not alleviated by confession. Quite the contrary, the neurotic felt more insecure after confession. The neurotic had to be shown God's love; the priest should never ridicule the neurotic. He had a psychiatric, not a moral problem.[30]

The theme of guilt figured less prominently in Judaism than in Christianity. Jewish theologians recognized the reality of guilt when man had transgressed God's law, and the importance of asking for forgiveness of sins from fellow men, and of atonement, particularly on Yom Kippur, the Day of Atonement. Psychological insights helped Jewish theologians understand how guilt feelings developed within the individual, and the necessity for self-acceptance and the acceptance of others, before one could free oneself of guilt.

Joshua Loth Liebman was opposed to a confession as a method of alleviating guilt, because he thought that atonement had a retarding effect on growth. He preferred psychoanalysis and the development of self-awareness, which entailed understanding without condemnation.[31]

Alexander Alan Steinbach stated in 1956 that guilt often resulted from depression. Depression was the result of loss, or the anticipation of loss. The inability to restore the loss resulted in anger, aggression, and guilt. Judaism taught that loss could occur as the result of sins, or because of some outside agency. The depression which resulted from the loss could be alleviated by prayer, repentance, and charity.[32] Steinbach concluded that Freud had shown that the mechanism of projection was the placing of anger which was really directed toward the self onto others.

David Kairys discussed special conflicts among the children of immigrant Jews in the United States in 1956. He alleged that the first generation Americans were raised to obey all the commandments of Orthodox Judaism. They then entered the non-Orthodox world which imposed fewer religious demands on the individual. The conflict between the values of childhood and those of adulthood caused many individuals to experience guilt feelings. Most Jews were able to successfully modify their consciences and achieve a compromise between the values of the old world and of the new, but some were not able to adapt and suffered from neurotic guilt or anxiety. A person with an overly strict conscience might deny himself the normal pleasures of life and might easily become prey to mental illness. Religious practices such as confession and penance could help relieve guilt feelings.[33]

Edward T. Sandrow proposed that guilt could also result from sin in the form of knowingly, perversely, or unknowingly defying God's laws. Sacrifice, prayer, and penance were the traditional religious aids for the alleviation of guilt. Sandrow noted that the forgiveness asked on Yom Kippur was asked of man, not of God, and man confessed his sins against himself, not against God. Man had to find acceptance within himself, and with his neighbor, before he could be at peace with God.

Sandrow thought that Jewish theology harmonized with the psychoanalytic insights of the neo-Freudians such as Sullivan, Horney, and Fromm. Man had to try to attain wholeness, self-acceptance, and the acceptance of others. Divine intervention or divine grace was not necessary.[34] God forgave man for sinning, when man accepted and forgave himself and others. Through forgiveness and acceptance of himself and of others, man could alleviate his guilt, although man was never entirely free from guilt. Participation in prayer rituals might also alleviate some guilt.[35]

In general theologians displayed a new sensitivity towards forms of neurotic guilt and the part it played in reactions to grief. Pleased that organized religion could help an individual overcome non-neurotic guilt feelings which were the result of real transgressions, Christian theologians were unanimous in praising the sacraments as aids in the reception of divine grace and forgiveness of sins. Jewish theologians mentioned penitential rituals in which man asked forgiveness of other men against whom he might have sinned and in turn received God's forgiveness. All theologians agreed that moderate guilt feelings were a sign of healthy relatedness between man and his environment.

Sin and Grief

Problems of anxiety and guilt were closely related to questions of sin. Protestant theologians insisted on the reality of sin. They realized that lack of a sense of sin or a moral sense, which might be due to a lack of relatedness to other individuals and the environment, could prevent a person from developing a sense of sin. Psychotherapy might be necessary before such a person could develop a sufficiently holistic self and moral sense to acquire a sense of sin. At the other extreme, a person who was suffering from neurotic guilt, or scrupulosity, might have an exaggerated or neurotic sense of sin.

Theologians advocated using the sacraments of the church, including confession, prayer, repentance, and divine forgiveness, to secure the remission of sins. They realized that self-acceptance and acceptance of others had to precede the true acceptance of divine forgiveness. The emphasis on the human relations in sin and forgiveness showed the influence of neo-Freudian psychology.

While Protestant theologians were concerned about the problem of scrupulosity, for them it was of less importance than for Catholics. An early comparison of sin and mental illness was offered by C. E. Barbour in 1930. He interpreted sin as a conscious or unconscious deviation from the Christian ideal. Neurotics sinned, but were guiltless. In addition, there were similarities between confession of sin and the formation of transference neuroses in psychiatry.[36] Love was essential for healing in both religion and psychiatry. This was an early statement of the importance of good object relations in the cure of sins and of neuroses.

While recognizing the effect of sin in fragmenting the personality, Ralph Higgins thought that there was a voluntary component in the commission of sin. He said that the individual deliberately embraced a regressive pattern when sinning, ignoring other factors in his environment; by doing so, the individual usurped God's place.[37] Edith H. Weigert, an existentialist psychologist, said in 1950 that psychology was against sin, but was not against the sinner.[38]

Ernest Bruder, a chaplain at St. Elizabeth's Hospital in Washington, D. C. and a leader in the field of clinical pastoral training, contended in 1952 that interpersonal relationships were the curative factor in the cure of sins. He explained that, in a theological sense, sin was separation from God and neighbors, and a separation in the personality of the sinner. Mental illness involved the same kind of separation. Therefore, sin was a type of mental illness, and psychology could provide the integrative and curative force for both.[39]

O. Hobart Mowrer, another existentialist psychoanalyst, was concerned about the problem of scrupulosity. He said that a balance had to be struck between seminaries which he said were now very Freudian in their orientation, and those who were unwilling to deal with the problem of neurotic guilt. A sound theology had to be psychologically sound in its handling of sin. He noted that a scrupulous person might be hiding a more serious sin. The cure for the problem of scrupulosity would be improved human relations, where he would receive good counter-transference from others.[40] The cure for sin, according to Mowrer, was not threats and admonitions, but re-socialization and re-integration of the personality, in a manner which would coincide with the neo-Freudian definition of the cure of neuroses. In 1963, O. H. Mowrer added that neuroses came from sin. The suppressed guilt over the sin was the cause of the neuroses.[41]

James A. Knight, who was active in the clinical training of ministers, said in 1962 that the psychiatric concept of the id as the location of base biological impulses did not differ from the theological doctrine of original sin, but a preacher who emphasized hell and damnation in his sermons did not love people. Such a preacher was himself full of hate and resentments.[42]

Catholics never doubted the existence of sin; man sinned because of his imperfect state. Sins had to be confessed and expiated through confession. The mentally ill remained responsible for their sins, because they possessed free will, but their guilt was lessened to the degree of their mental illness.

Catholics were concerned about the problem of scrupulosity, which involved neurotic guilt and the confession of imaginary sins. Through the influence of psychology, Catholics realized that scrupulosity was a psychiatric problem which the priest should refer to a psychotherapist. The priest should discourage the obsessive confession of sins. A person who suffered from scrupulosity needed a priest in the confessional, and needed a psychoanalyst to help him overcome his scrupulosity.[43]

Odenwald and VanderVeldt asserted that a scrupulous person was in some cases hiding other sins. In other instances, it might be a sign of egotism. The priest had to decide when a referral to a psychotherapist was necessary, and he had to deal with all aspects of sin as moral matters. The priest and the psychiatrist should agree on a definition of sin, so that a patient suffering from scrupulosity would not become further confused in the course of treatment.[44]

Jewish views about the nature of sin were affected by Freudian and neo-Freudian psychology. Jewish writers said that the sinner was mentally ill, and that an improvement in interpersonal relations of the sinner was the best way to secure the remission of sins.

Man was not inherently sinful, according to traditional Jewish theology. Judaism did not accept the doctrine of original sin, and did not recognize any insurmountable impediment between man and perfection. Thus Jewish theology recognized the existence of sin, but sin was not a major theme in Jewish thought. Jewish writers recognized that the problem of scrupulosity was a mental health problem, but did not consider it a major one.

Henry Enoch Kagan alleged that the only non-Jewish thought in Freud's writing was his statement that man was sinful. There was no doubt that sin existed, and when misdeeds had occurred, a sense of guilt and sin was a sign of mental health.[45]

According to Jewish theology, man was born with a clean soul, and with the potential for leading a life without sin. Man was good, life was good, and man should enjoy it fully. Man could attain perfection. Jewish theologians found Sullivan's theories particularly attractive, because Sullivan had said that man was born whole, with an unblemished ego. Bad object relations caused ego splitting in man, and a resultant loss of wholeness and inability to relate to others.

Edward T. Sandrow insisted that by the Jewish tradition, to sin was to knowingly, perversely, or innocently violate God's law. The greatest

sin that man could commit was to stifle or deprecate one's own self.
Evidence of sinfulness in Judaism was demonstrating lack of respect for
the teachings of the Bible and the Talmud. Other evidence of sin were
excessive materialism and the stifling of the spiritual self. Sin triumphed
when man stopped himself from loving himself and fellow man.
Sandrow added that traditional Jewish literature taught that sin was folly
or, in modern terminology, mental illness. The mentally healthy person
would be less likely to sin.[46] Theologians continued to re-affirm the
existence of sin. Reactions to sin, much like reactions to guilt, could be
healthy or unhealthy. Christian ministers agreed that the sacraments of
the church including confession, penitence and prayer were effective in
securing divine forgiveness of sins and the elimination of guilt feelings.
Excessive feelings of sinfulness gained new recognition as psychological
not religious. Judaism continued to differ from Christianity in its view
about the absence of original sin, while theologians gained a new
understanding of the neurotic element in exaggerated feelings of
sinfulness, and of the idea that the sinner was a sick rather than an evil
person.

Theologians from Protestantism, Catholicism, and Judaism accepted
the description of grief given by Freud in *Mourning and Melancholia*[47]
and the theories of the neo-Freudians about the importance of forming
new interpersonal relations in order to fill the void left by the inter-
ruption of interpersonal relations which resulted from bereavement.

Psychoanalytic theories about the nature of grief were of great help
to pastors, who were often called upon to comfort the bereaved. Pastors
developed a deeper understanding of the dynamics of grief, and of the
role that real and neurotic guilt played in the work that an individual
had to do to overcome grief. It was the job of the pastor to discover the
emotional state of the bereaved, and help them do the mental work
which was necessary before they could overcome their grief.

In 1950, William F. Rogers said that grief was the result of broken
interpersonal relationships. The grief-stricken person had many intense
social needs, whose fulfillment would help compensate the bereaved for
the lost relationship.[48] The editors of *Pastoral Psychology* advised pastors
on comforting the bereaved in cases of suicide. Since the cause of
suicide was often unknown, it was best to see it as the end of a fatal
illness, but the reality of the loss needed to be acknowledged.[49]

Erich Lindeman described the syndrome which was associated with
acute grief. He found that it had both psychological and somatic
importance; it might appear immediately after a crisis, or it might be
exaggerated if delayed. By appropriate counseling techniques, exaggerated
grief could be converted into normal grief, which then could be

overcome. Religious workers could help the bereaved overcome guilt which the bereaved might feel towards the deceased by offering them the sacraments, but religious comfort alone was not enough. Real grief work had to take place, which involved dissolving the bonds with the deceased, readjusting to the environment and forming new relationships which could in part compensate for the loss of the deceased.[50]

Psychoanalytic understanding of the dynamics of dying could also help the pastor work with the terminally ill. Psychotherapy could bring about greater self-acceptance and existential reconciliation to the dying, so that the dying person would not feel that his life had been wasted.[51]

William Rogers declared that grief was not the result of what happened to the deceased, but rather what happened to the bereaved. A mature bereaved person who was free of neurotic ties to the deceased, and who had strong relationships with other family members and friends, could stand the loss better, and would have less need of the clergy-man, than a person with more neurotic ties to the deceased and fewer supportive relationships.[52]

Catholic theologians devoted little attention to the problem of grief. The traditional Catholic belief in God and in an afterlife was the main support for the bereaved, augmented by the social aspects of the wake. The problem of grief was not discussed.

Jewish writers, who tried to demonstrate that psychology and religion were compatible, were delighted to point out that Jewish mourning and funeral practices closely paralleled the types of grief work which psychologists said were necessary for an individual to overcome a bereavement.

In 1946, Joshua Loth Liebman said it was necessary to express, rather than to contain, the emotions associated with grief, and partially to replace the ties to the dead with bonds to other individuals. He noted that guilt was part of the emotions which were associated with bereavement.

Traditional Jewish practices of burial and mourning gave the bereaved an excellent opportunity to work out their grief. Among these practices was the rapid burial, within twenty-four hours, of the unembalmed body dressed in a simple white shroud and placed in a plain casket. The traditional philosophy was that the body was dust and must return to dust as rapidly as possible through natural processes. The bereaved then returned home for a meal which was to be prepared by neighbors. They observed seven days of *shiva* or full mourning, during which time friends and family were to visit them, bringing food. The remainder of the first month consisted of days of semi-mourning, during which the bereaved gradually rebuilt his relationships with others. There were eleven more months of more gradual rebuilding. Excessive mourning was forbidden by Judaism.

Jewish mourning and burial practices were considered to be psychologically valid, because the rapid and simple burial led to a prompt acceptance of the death, and the rapid breaking of the bond of human relations. Once the loss was accepted, the bereaved could turn his attention to rebuilding the bonds with other people, in order to mitigate the loss. The gradual emergence from deep mourning was thought to give the person time to overcome any guilt, resentment, or anger which he might feel towards the deceased.[53]

Simon Noveck agreed completely with Liebman, and he added that appropriate conversation with the bereaved included reviewing the satisfying relationship that the bereaved or others had enjoyed with the deceased. The Jewish prayer for the dead and the memorial services were affirmations of life rather than lamentations, which would help draw the attention of the bereaved to the continuation of life. In addition, they were a reaffirmation of faith and trust in God. Faith in immortality was another source of comfort. The Jewish belief was that the soul was immortal; it also lived on through the memory of the good deeds the person had performed during his lifetime.[54]

Jack D. Spiro agreed with the statements of Noveck and Liebman concerning the compatibility of Jewish mourning practices and psychological insights about the nature of mourning with the way in which grief work was accomplished. He noted that modern society had made it more difficult for adequate grief work to occur, because of customs which served to deny death, and the pressure of time, which limited the period spent in mourning.[55]

Thus, the Protestant response to the psychological analysis of grief was to explain the stages through which a mourner passed and the relationship of his general state of mental health to his reaction to grief. The main objective of theologians was to insure that pastoral counseling of mourners would be psychologically sound. Jewish writers seemed satisfied that traditional Jewish mourning practices were psychologically valid and in this case, traditional practices received confirmation from psychology. Catholic theologians did not explore the problem.

Love, Forgiveness and Salvation

Neo-Freudian theories about the importance of good object relations for the establishment and maintenance of mental health caused some Protestant pastors to place more emphasis on the emotion of love. Self-healing and reunification of self could only be accomplished through love of self. Love of self and of one's fellow men had to precede love of God and the acceptance of God's love and forgiveness. Obedience to God's laws should proceed out of love, not from fear of divine punishment. Protestants differentiated between Christian love, called *agape*, and sexual or erotic love, called *eros*. They considered *eros* to be divisive and anti-Christian. They emphasized the role of *agape* in healing and in bringing men together in an anxious, war-torn world.

Edith Weigert, an existentialist psychologist, said that both psychiatry and religion were concerned with love which brought peace and integrity to the human soul. Fear and hate had the opposite effect; they were paralyzing defense reactions which caused guilt and isolation, while religious faith was capable of transcending fear and was rooted in love. Love had to be spontaneous and could overcome every person's isolation.[56]

Self-love was necessary before love of others would be possible, declared Paul Johnson in 1951. He was influenced by neo-Freudian concepts about the importance of love, and declared that parental rejection turned children into neurotics and criminals who could not work with others because they could not accept themselves.[57] Johnson thought in 1956 that love was the best teacher and the heart of all religion.[58]

Catholic theologians were favorable to neo-Freudian theories about the necessity of self-acceptance and the acceptance of others, but Odenwald and VanderVeldt retained the traditional Christian formulation that man's first duty was to love God. One should also love one's neighbor as well as one loved oneself. This formulation was at variance with Freudian thought. Although obedience through love of God was preferable to obedience through fear, obedience to the teachings of the Church took precedence over the doctrine of love in most Catholic writings.[59]

All the Jews writing about psychology and religion stressed the importance of love of self and self-acceptance before love and acceptance of others was possible. They also said that self-love and respect was part of traditional Jewish thought. Man was made in God's image and was good, as was life and the world. Life was to be enjoyed, and love was part of enjoyment. Despite the acceptance of the importance of love of self and of others as a manifestation and prelude to love of God, love was not a major theme in Jewish thought. Ruth Levy emphasized the importance of love. She asserted that psychiatry offered a method of healing: working towards greater feelings of security through both teaching and giving love.[60] According to theories of Sullivan and

Horney, it was necessary to accept and like one's self before one could accept and love others.

Theologians of all faiths placed new emphasis on self-love and self-acceptance as preludes to the love and acceptance of others and finally of God. Protestant theologians were in part reaffirming the traditional concept of *agape*, but with a new urgency which seemed to be required by the hostilities of the 1940s and the 1950s. Brotherly love was now necessary for the survival of mankind. Reform Jewish theologians drew from traditional Jewish sources to bring theology into line with psychological practice. Catholic theologians acknowledged the importance of self-love but retained the traditional formulation of love of God as primary, with brotherly love and self-love following as corollaries, in that order.

Forgiveness remained an important concept in Protestant theology. The influence of neo-Freudian psychology promoted increased stress on the forgiveness of one's self as a prerequisite for the forgiveness of others and the acceptance of divine forgiveness in that order. This represented a shift in emphasis in Protestant theology rather than a new departure. For example, Paul E. Johnson said in 1951 that the attainment of insight or self-understanding preceded forgiveness, while forgiveness enabled people to grow.[61] John Dolard and Neale E. Miller said that forgiveness reduced the sense of human isolation and indicated acceptance.[62]

Donald S. Arbuckle announced that client-centered therapy would be Christian and God-centered if God was seen as loving and forgiving. He thought that the concept of the wrathful or avenging God was inappropriate in the Christian therapeutic setting. Acceptance and forgiveness on the part of the therapist would enable the individual to stop rejecting himself.[63] Aleck Dodd agreed that acceptance of God's forgiveness was part of man's trusting surrender to a loving God. He thought that through the surrender to a forgiving God, man could become whole.[64]

Forgiveness was not a major theme in Jewish modern thought. Jewish formulations of forgiveness were affected by Freudian psychology to the extent that Jewish theologians realized that forgiveness of self and of others had to precede the acceptance of God's forgiveness.[65]

The Catholic view of divine forgiveness was not greatly changed by psychoanalytic insights, beyond the increased emphasis which was placed upon the importance of love in man's relationship with God. The traditional view of forgiveness prevailed, which was that the penitent received God's forgiveness from the priest after the confession of sins.

The ultimate aim of Protestant pastoral counseling remained salvation. The change caused by the acceptance of neo-Freudian concepts of the nature of man was the realization that the acceptance of God's forgiveness and the acceptance of Christ as the Savior could only come after self-acceptance and the acceptance of fellow men.

Wilfred Daim explained the meaning of the Freudian term "fixation." He said that it was the idolization of an object from childhood. Worldly fixations had to be overcome and worldly conflicts healed before a person could focus on God as the true absolute, and then salvation could be achieved.[66]

Salvation was the aim of all Catholic counseling. There was no significant change from the traditional way of achieving salvation through prayer, the sacraments and following the teachings of the Church.

Salvation was not a concept which was stressed in Judaism. Jewish theology postulated eternal life, but was much more vague about the method of attainment, beyond obeying God's laws and doing the 613 *mitzvot* which were required of a Jew.

Mysticism, Worship and Conversion

Mysticism had not been an area of great concern to Protestant theologians in the twentieth century. Since mysticism remained outside the mainstream of religious practice, there had been little effort to assimilate psychoanalytic concepts into the theology of mysticism.

Anton T. Boisen, a pioneer in the clinical training movement, was interested in similarities between certain forms of mental illness and mystical experiences. He said in 1939 that the impact of mystical experience on some people was similar to the impact of mental illness.[67] In 1952, he reported on studies of college and theological students and male mental patients who had had mystical experiences in which they identified with Jesus.[68]

In 1965, D. H. Salman discussed the psychology of religious experience. Saying that regression provided the link between mystical states and psychoses, he called psychosis a pressured withdrawal, often with a complete return. The mystical state was one of controlled withdrawal and return, a death and rebirth.[69]

Catholic writers had a long record of interest in studying the lives of mystical saints like St. Teresa of Avila. Progressives sought to do this in the light of modern psychology, but devout Catholics viewed the mystical experiences of saints as evidence of divine grace and not really appropriate material for psychological analysis. Mysticism had not been a major strain of Catholic thought since the middle ages and could not be considered a major concern of modern day theologians.

Mysticism had been a very minor concern and one often suppressed by religious leaders in Judaism. It retained only esoteric interest for Jewish scholars.

Ministers realized that the worship service could be utilized to promote individual growth and to improve group dynamics. Alfred Haas believed that the worship service could relieve egocentricity and isolation and could provide a form of group therapy. Hymns could be used to focus attention outside the self, bring comfort through words and music, reduce anxiety and alleviate guilt. The pastor, therefore, should choose hymns with care. Hymns should encourage social responsibility, not immaturity and dependency or infantile regression.[70]

The sermon too should make the listener feel liked, wanted, and secure. Criticism should be limited. The goals and standards of parishioners should be respected even if they did not measure up to those of the pastor. The aim of the sermon was to make people feel independent, responsible, and trustworthy.[71] A minister's style of preaching also depended upon his personality. Schizoid and paranoid styles of preaching were the most harmful.[72]

Worship services could be an aid in the treatment of a person receiving psychiatric treatment at home. The minister should encourage a positive attitude towards the mentally ill, but care had to be taken to make the services as socially-oriented and purposeful as possible. Worship services were developed in a period when Protestantism placed greater stress on man's dependence on God than is considered to be mentally healthy today.[73]

There was no discussion of Catholic liturgy in relation to psychoanalytic concepts during the time period included in this study. There have been many changes in Catholic liturgical practices since the Second Vatican Council ended in 1965. Many of these changes were designed to increase the participation of the worshipper; for example, the new method of receiving holy communion.

Nor was there discussion of psychology and liturgical practices in the relevant Jewish literature. Patterns of Orthodox worship remained unchanged. There had been some increased interest in lay participation in worship services among Reform Jews and slightly less among Conservative Jews.

Protestant theologians continued to view conversion experiences as evidence of the individual's reorienting his life towards God. Some acknowledged that conversion experience could be regressive as well as progressive, although the desirability of the experience seemed to overshadow the inherent dangers.

The influence of Freudian psychology could be seen in the acknowledgment of the regressive nature of some conversion experiences, and the influence of neo-Freudian psychology in the criteria drawn by Boisen for evaluating whether a conversion experience was a genuine turning toward God or a symptom of mental illness.

Anton T. Boisen said in 1928 that recovery from mental illness was similar to a conversion experience, because both involved a reorganization of the personality.[74] In 1936 he explored the relationship between acute functional mental illness and sudden changes in character of Christian patriarchs like Saul of Tarsus or George Fox. He suggested that some mental disorders and conversions such as St. Paul's conversion were attempts at reorganization of the personality, which, when unsuccessful, led to mental illness. Religious workers working with the mentally ill could help them have a conversion experience which would lead to a successful reorganization of personality and to mental health.

Boisen believed that mental illness was a reaction to the environment rather than a physical disease. He accepted the Gestalt theory of psychology that the whole was greater than the sum of its parts. Feelings that one's life was a failure might precipitate mental illness. A conversion experience might bring new harmony to the individual. Religious workers should conduct services in mental hospitals in which the patient could participate, and chaplains should participate in the treatment of mental patients to facilitate a conversion experience.[75]

Boisen described the case history of a neurotic who had been freed from his neurotic guilt, resulting from sexual drives, when he underwent a conversion experience and experienced God's forgiveness. He stressed that the conversion was brought about by a relationship of love between the therapist and the patient.[76]

In 1950, Harry M. Tiebout examined the process of conversion. He said that a person who experienced conversion lost his "tense, aggressive, demanding, isolated conscience-ridden self" to become a more "relaxed," "realistic" person who was more at home in the world. The key element in the personality change was surrender of the ego to God on the unconscious level. Surrender and catharsis produced the sensation of feeling better, and if the surrender continued, would cause the maintenance of the improved state of mind.[77] A conversion experience of a child was a sudden or gradual change in primordial impulses, although the nature of the power which caused the change was difficult for the child to understand.[78]

According to Carl Christensen, adolescent conversion experiences were different. They reflected an intra-psychic conflict involving anxiety and guilt and a need for commitment. He reviewed traditional Protestant definitions of conversion, formulated by pre-Freudian psychologists of religion. Freud had said that a conversion experience represented an attempt to resolve the Oedipal conflict of the individual. Christensen also referred to Salzman, a neo-Freudian psychiatrist, who was interested in pastoral psychology and who viewed the conversion experience as part of the process of adaptation to adult life. He said that there were two types of conversion experiences. One was progressive and maturational; the other was regressive or psycho-pathological. In the latter, Salzman agreed that Freud's explanation was valid.

Salzman thought that a conversion experience could be resolved in one of four ways. There could be reintegration of the ego at a new level of maturity, a reintegration at the previous level, a reintegration at a lower level of functioning, or a failure of the ego to be reintegrated at all.[79]

In 1961 Anton Boisen asserted that most psychiatrists considered any patient who heard voices to be schizophrenic. Boisen, however, felt that the experience of mental patients in hearing voices was identical with voices heard by those having a religious experience which led to greater creativity. Whether the voices were a sign of personal disorganization or a religious "call" depended upon whether the individual was able to perform according to normal standards. The individual had to accept a competent religious counselor and abide by the social standards of some accepted group. The convert would also have to accept the veracity of the call. In addition, he would be judged on future behavior and on his tolerance for frustration.[80] Thus, Boisen evaluated a conversion experience empirically in terms of an individual's religious orientation and ability to relate to his environment.

A comparable situation was identified by Harry M. Tiebout in the experience of an alcoholic when he hit bottom. Without surrender of the ego as in a conversion experience, an alcoholic could hit bottom many times without any significant change in his behavior. Tiebout thought that "ego reduction" was the essential element in a conversion experience. The individual had to surrender his all-powerful ego and admit the existence of a higher power. Tiebout was using the term ego in a neo-Freudian sense. In Freudian terminology, the individual would have to be less narcissistic.[81]

In 1965, Earl H. Furgeson claimed that with little development in the field of psychology and religion, the retrogressive nature of some conversion experiences had to be acknowledged. Not all conversion experiences, whether sudden or gradual, resulted in regeneration of the personality.[82]

Conversion experiences were not as important in Catholic theology as in Protestant, which had more evangelical elements. The surrender to God was acknowledged, but conversion experiences were discussed in terms of manifestations of divine grace rather than in psychoanalytic terms.

Nor were conversion experiences which entailed a turning towards God very common in modern Judaism. Jewish theologians were aware of Freudian theories about the regressive nature of a conversion experience and the inherent dangers, and they were aware that a return to the community of Judaism held within it the possibility for improved object relations.

Milton R. Saperstein discussed the type of religious conversion which led to renewed interest in Judaism. He did not deal with religious conversions which resulted in a change of religion. In his view some Jews returned to more Orthodox religious practices as a rebellion against their parents, who had dropped most of their religious identification in the process of acculturation.

Conversion experiences represented a movement to the past. They could be beneficial. They tended to be authoritarian and regressive or harmful to the individual. A sense of helplessness and surrender to God was felt. There might also be a sense of obedience and atonement and of almost complete martyrdom of the person, and a mystical or symbolic loss of body boundaries. There might be a loss of identity, or hallucination might be experienced. The convert might find a new sense of peace as he accepted an explanation of the world order which was held by his coreligionists, and might experience a sense of tradition and returning to the past. He might feel a new appreciation of the world.

Saperstein concluded that in humanistic Judaism the convert would probably enjoy improved interpersonal relations, because most aspects of Jewish life and prayer were group activities and stressed human relations. A religious experience would entail an honest return to the good aspects of one's "personal past," to one's ethnic background, and to a humanistic outlook with a hopeful attitude toward the future.[83]

Protestant and Jewish theologians examined conversion experiences very closely, applying psychological insights and gathering empirical evidence to determine whether a religious conversion or a mental breakdown had occurred. This was another attempt to make theology psychologically valid.

Sex

Protestant theology reflected the new appreciation of the importance of accepting normal mature sexuality, as did the rest of American culture. Although theologians rejected Freud's biological theory that the sex instinct and sexual energies provided the motivation for all human behavior, they did accept neo-Freudian theories that sexual behavior was part of all interpersonal relations. Freud accomplished the partial overthrow of Victorian repression of sexuality. All forms of sexual behavior, such as masturbation and mature sexuality, were judged by their effect upon the development of sound interpersonal relations rather than on the basis of biblical injunctions against fornication, masturbation, or homosexuality.

Protestant theologians continued to teach that the proper expression of sexual desires was within marriage. They did not approve of extra-marital sex, which they considered to be immoral and to present a danger to society.

There was a new appreciation of the sexuality of women and a feeling that the preference for asceticism expressed by St. Paul, Luther, and Calvin might not contain a healthy attitude towards sexuality. Freud's theoretical formulations concerning penis envy among women, and the existence and the formulation of the Oedipus complex were seen as reflections of the male-dominated Victorian society in which he lived, rather than as expressing a universal norm. Freud's theory of infant sexuality was almost completely rejected. Thus, D. Yellowless in 1930 charged that St. Paul's views on the origin of sin, as well as his attitude towards his body and towards women, were repressive and should be changed.[84]

J. R. Oliver recognized that marital maladjustment presented a pastoral problem for clergymen. He conceded that each individual had homo-erotic and hetero-erotic tendencies and the dominance of each tendency in each individual determined his sexual orientation. Auto-eroticism was an immature state of sexual development and was undesirable. Oliver thought that religious faith and practice could help cure sexual maladjustments. He alleged that both Jesus and psychiatrists in effect had said that an individual must lose his fixations, including his sexual fixations, in order to be well.[85]

Anton Boisen wrote in 1942 about a boy who had a conversion experience after suffering from acute anxiety and guilt because he masturbated. Boisen saw the problem of masturbation in terms of a breakdown in interpersonal relations. He said that through psychotherapy the boy stopped masturbating and was able to form better social relations which ended his isolation. Boisen thought that through religious faith and hope the boy could be helped to deal with his frailties.[86]

Sylvanus Duvall agreed in 1952 that sexual morality was a part of all human behavior and, therefore, could not be considered as a private matter. He accepted the Christian view of man as basically spiritual, with sexual fulfillment being of lesser importance.[87]

Joseph Fletcher tried to develop a moral philosophy of sexual standards in 1953. He criticized Freud for failing to relate sexual behavior to culture, and for considering people as isolated personalities who were internally motivated by conflicting drives from the id, ego, and superego. He insisted that even Freud's followers, including Karen Horney and Abraham Kardiner, had rejected Freud's formulation of the origins of sexual behavior. Sexual behavior was to be understood in terms of interpersonal relations and interactions. Character governed sexual behavior, not the reverse. A person's values and philosophy determined how he satisfied his sexual desires. Various neurotic forms of behavior including sadism, selfishness, and exploitation were evidenced in sexual behavior. Psychiatrists agreed that people who treated sex as an end in itself were sick, said Fletcher. A moral philosophy of sex would be based upon mutually supportive interpersonal relations between sexual partners and would encourage their personal and societal integration.[88]

Ashley Montagu, a noted anthropologist, criticized Freud's theory of sexuality for its inadequate treatment of the role of women. He praised Freud's psychological system as the best known to man. Montagu contended that Freud never understood the relationship between mother and child or between lovers. He questioned the concepts of penis envy, the Oedipus complex, the destructive urges, and the narcissistic stage as a normal phase of development. Montagu preferred the formulation of Ian Suttie, an English psychoanalyst who named love as the organizing force in the personality. He thought that love and sex were drives which aimed at the preservation of life.[89]

Karl Menninger announced in 1954 that the Kinsey Report[90] confirmed Freud's theory that civilized man paid for the progress of civilization by the suppression of his instincts and the development of his inhibitions.[91]

Seward Hiltner agreed in 1953 that sexual fulfillment was a deep and moving experience that led the mature adult to greater love of his partner and to improved interpersonal relationships, personal integration, and the assumption of social responsibility. Gothard Booth said that masturbation was the sign of the need for closeness with another person rather than a symptom of the need for sexual intercourse. When masturbation was compulsive it was a psychological problem; in other cases, masturbation acted as a safety valve for the release of sexual tensions. Treatment of compulsive masturbation treated the underlying organic or psychological problem.[92]

William Cole traced and explained the origin and development of Christian attitudes toward sex. He argued that the Greek and Jewish philosophies of sex were in conflict. Greek thought considered mind and body as a duality while Jewish thought considered sex as a natural part of man's existence which could not and should not be repressed. Then Luther anticipated Freud in recognizing the complex aspect of the sexual drive. Luther and Freud differed in that Luther regarded sex as sinful while Freud considered it a natural instinct. Cole noted that both Freud and Luther accepted sex in marriage but did not enjoy it.[93]

Including a survey of contemporary Protestant attitudes toward sex — for instance, the approval of sex education and the acceptance of sex within marriage as something good — he also surveyed the belief that all men were lustful, that contraception was acceptable, and that not all people made suitable marriage partners. In addition, the emancipation of women had changed notions about female sexuality and had raised questions about female satisfaction which had not yet been satisfactorily answered, although dual standards of sexual behavior for men and women still existed.

Protestant acceptance of the world entailed acceptance of human sexuality, and the primary goal of sexual relations was the furtherance of interpersonal relations, not procreation. Masturbation was permissible if it was not excessive and did not eliminate the need for interpersonal relations. No man was free from sin, anxiety, or hostility.[94]

Adolf Meyer, a psychoanalyst, said that repression of the sex instinct was not always bad; when it led to the establishment of families, it was good. Repression, too, could be normal or abnormal. Normal repression was necessary for the establishment of society.[95]

Lester Kirkendull disapproved of pre-marital sexual relationships because they seldom furthered human relations.[96] Norman C. Morgan said that it was easy for his clients to accept the urgency of the sex drive as being similar to hunger or fatigue but different in that it could be expressed in a variety of ways, both healthy and unhealthy. Masturbation was not the best way to express the sex drive because it did not further interpersonal relations.[97]

Vere Loper said in 1957 that any abnormal expression of sexuality, whether it was puritanism or licentiousness, endangered the maintenance of family life.[98]

D. C. McClelland attributed Freud's attitude towards sex to Freud's being Jewish. McClelland said that Freud denied that psychoanalysis was exclusively Jewish because of prevalent anti-Semitism during Freud's lifetime. McClelland said that the Old Testament contained many discussions of sex.[99]

Milton J. Huber advocated counseling the single woman that she sublimate her sex drive and find non-sexual outlets for her energies, and that she accept her unmarried state.[100] Acceptance of being single would be part of self-acceptance, but sublimation of the sex drive was advised because extra-marital sexual relations were unacceptable.

Carroll A. Wise noted that ministers were called upon to do a great deal of marriage counseling. He advocated the use of testing, such as the Sex Knowledge Inventory Test, and the use of dynamic psychology and techniques of pastoral counseling and marital counseling.[101]

Thomas Bingham said in 1960 that a pastor should accept the confession of masturbation without displaying approval or disapproval, and he should definitely not exaggerate the evil consequences of masturbation. Stressing the evils of masturbation would just increase the individual's feelings of guilt and anxiety without assisting him in his need to improve his interpersonal relations.[102]

Gothard Booth expressed similar thoughts to those of Bingham in 1961. He said that compulsive masturbation was not a sexual problem but a social problem. The real problem was that parents or teachers sometimes encouraged children to develop guilt feelings about normal masturbation. Thomas Bingham added that the Bible never spoke against masturbation, but that sexual activities which increased human isolation were undesirable.[103] Mature heterosexual relations had their place within the marital relationship. Sex education was necessary in order for children to develop healthy attitudes towards sex. Odenwald and VanderVeldt thought that children should be told "where babies came from" and that sex education should be completed before the individual was twenty-one years old.[104] They also said that immaturity was the most common cause of divorce, followed by economic problems or difficulties.[105]

Masturbation was clearly a mortal sin in an adult, although it was normal in a child or in an adolescent. Sex education, self-control, and self-discipline were the proper ways to discourage the practice. Once masturbation became compulsive in an adult, it was very difficult to cure. Masturbation in adults could sometimes cause mental illness, because it caused conflicts within the individual. Masturbation was a mortal sin in a healthy person. They reported that priests and psychotherapists had achieved only moderate success in treating homosexuals, of whom they recommended charitable understanding.[106]

The only way that psychoanalytic insights could be said to have influenced the Catholic view of masturbation was that it would be considered as less than a mortal sin in a neurotic, and that it was considered advisable to give a good education about sexual matters, rather than scare stories designed to stop the practice by frightening the individual.[107] Another change was increased stress on the importance of sexuality within marriage as part of the marital relationship in which the members displayed love and respect for one another.

Traditional Judaism had always accepted man's sexuality as an integral part of his being. Therefore, psychoanalytic concepts caused little change in Jewish thinking. Extramarital sex was not accepted because it was seen as presenting a danger to the family and to society. Although there was no discussion in the relevant literature, it is reasonable to assume that in Reform and Conservative Judaism, masturbation and homosexuality were viewed as psychological problems rather than as sins.

In the twentieth century, people relaxed their standards of sexual morality, and theologians became aware of the importance of the expression of mature sexuality. Liberalized views on sexual morality reflected, therefore, an attempt to make theology psychologically valid and contained some unavoidable concessions to changes in moral standards. Theologians remained most concerned that sexuality further interpersonal relations and that the structure of the family be preserved. Catholic and Orthodox Jewish sexual standards changed least.

Conclusion

The three major religious groups altered their theological concepts to different extents. The greatest changes occurred in theologically progressive Protestant denominations and in Reform Judaism. Orthodox Judaism remained almost completely unaffected, and Catholicism was slow to respond, modifying only their most extreme positions.

Naturally, religionists were happiest when they discovered that traditional religious practices were psychologically valid. The concurrence of Protestant and to some extent Jewish emphasis on fellowship and *agape* as aids to mental health with the neo-Freudian emphasis on interpersonal or object relations was a case in point. Similarly, traditional Jewish mourning practices seemed, to reform theologians, to be psychologically valid. In other cases theologians were willing to give questionable emphasis to citations of ancient sources to prove that traditional thought was valid in terms of modern psychology. Jewish theologians seemed especially prone to this type of endeavor although theologians from all three groups were guilty to some extent.

In other areas psychology had offered new interpretations of man's behavior which made some traditional forms of religious behavior seem less desirable. Recognition of the problems of neurotic guilt and of scrupulosity, and of the total lack of guilt as indicative of mental illness represent areas where theology deliberately strove to incorporate psychology in order to further mental health. Another important change was the stress on the necessity of self-love and self-acceptance which had to precede love of others and of God. This was accompanied by a general elevation of the worshipper from a debased sinner to a human capable of great love and joyful striving to fulfill God's commandments, who could accept God's forgiveness as the culmination of his efforts to love and to accept himself, his fellow man and God. Catholics retained the traditional formulation of love of God as primary followed by love of others at the same intensity as self-love. In addition, theologians no longer greeted all conversion experiences with a resounding hallelujah. Instead, they looked for empirical evidence in the subsequent behavior of the convert as to whether he was experiencing divine grace or mental illness. In other cases theologians seemed to rationalize existing changes. More relaxed sexual attitudes were examples of this kind of change.

Religious Uses of Psychology

The impact of Freudian varieties of psychology upon religious theory, that is upon theological ideas, was substantial, although its exact extent is hard to measure. This is a common situation in the history of ideas. But when one turns to the application of Freudian psychology to religious practice, any doubts of the substantial quality of Freudian influence fade close to the vanishing point. The administration of religion expressed in hierarchy, priesthood and lay relations found Freudian techniques and practices well worth borrowing, though usually with modifications. It is the purpose of this chapter to trace those uses of psychology by organized religion, which centered in the areas in ministerial training, pastoral counseling of individuals, and congregational or group techniques.

The Clinical Training of Ministers

Probably the greatest impact of psychology on religion occurred in the training of ministers for their pastoral duties. Liberal Protestantism was affected the most. However, all seminary curricula bear witness to the flood of new courses of a psychological nature which drastically altered pastoral education. Courses in pastoral theology became programs in clinical training based upon a psychological model. The philosophy of ministers doing pastoral counseling changed to resemble that of clinical psychologists, and ministers worked as part of community health teams.

Religious institutions also made extensive use of testing procedures to screen seminarians so that those who were deemed unfit for the ministry might be denied admission. Psychological tests were used also to evaluate the success of religious education programs in changing attitudes and beliefs and to measure attitudes among religious and non-religious people.

The greatest impact of Freudian psychology in American Protestantism was the change in the role and the education of the pastor. Traditionally a minister was an authoritarian, judgmental but kindly interpreter of moral law who was a sympathetic listener and dispenser of comfort and forgiveness through the sacraments of the church. A new role was now held up for emulation—the trained counselor who based his contacts with parishioners upon the principles of psychotherapy. The clinically trained pastor might still give comfort through the sacraments of the church. But, he now realized that the parishioner had to be reconciled with himself and with his fellow man before comfort, divine forgiveness, and reconciliation could be truly accepted.

Seminary education changed more specifically. Psychology first entered the seminaries through courses in psychology of religion. This was before Freudian concepts were widely known or accepted in the United States. In the early 1900s, under the influence of William James and James Starbuck, the Hartford School of Religious Pedagogy, which was affiliated with the Hartford Theological Seminary, began to offer courses in psychology of religion. Courses in psychology of religion slowly proliferated in progressive seminaries in the Northeastern United States, often under the aegis of the department of religious education.[1]

Psychology of religion had spread to the midwestern United States by 1927. A course entitled "Types of Religious Experiences and Personality Disorders" was offered at the Chicago Theological School, but the expansion rate of such courses continued to be slow for some time.

By 1930, depth psychology was taught as part of clinical training programs. Philip Guiles, the Director of the Council for Clinical Training of Theological Students, gave a course entitled "Clinical Psychological and Pastoral Work" and another called "Personal Counseling." These courses were combined with training internships in hospitals.

After 1932 there was a great increase in the number of course offerings in clinical pastoral training. Dissatisfaction with traditional training courses and a desire on the part of ministers to be able to ease their parishioners' anxiety led to the change in pastoral education. Pastoral training courses in combination with institutional internships were often given during the summer.

In addition to offerings in applied psychology, seminaries introduced courses in psychology in combination with supervised clinical training internships which were designed to train institutional chaplains. Clinically trained ministers first practiced among the sick in mental, general, and veterans' hospitals and among prisoners. The first practitioners of this new ministry often had experienced mental illness themselves. They were interested in studying Freudian psychology in order to find better insights into man's nature. They studied techniques of counseling which could ultimately bring man closer to God, and they hoped to become more effective counselors who gained more satisfaction from their work.[2]

However, the leaders of the movement worked hard at defining what they considered to be the unique role of the clinically trained pastoral counselor in terms acceptable to a wide range of denominations. The movement always lacked solid financial support because no denomination felt a strong responsibility for its growth and survival. They also tried to establish clinical and educational criteria for pastoral counselors, hoping to insure that such practitioners were adequately trained for the difficult jobs they were undertaking and that they would gain acceptance as part of clinically trained mental health teams.

The idea of clinical pastoral training was first set forth in 1913 at the General Convention of the Protestant Episcopal Church by the Rev. William Palmer Ladd who later became Dean of Berkeley Divinity School in New Haven, Connecticut.[3] In 1922, William S. Keller of Cincinnati, a doctor of medicine, agreed to supervise some seminarians who served as chaplains in comunity service organizations; next year the Cincinnati Summer School for the clinical training of seminarians was opened. In 1936, the Reverend Joseph F. Fletcher founded the Graduate School for Applied Religion of the Episcopal Church at Cambridge, Massachusetts. He was interested in providing a post-graduate year of study for seminarians during which they would receive clinical training by serving as interns in an institution.

Anton T. Boisen, an Episcopal minister, was considered to be the father of the clinical training movement. Early in his career Boisen suffered from bouts of mental illness which required hospitalization. After recovery Boisen studied at the Harvard Divinity School and at Andover Theological Seminary. Also, Boisen was influenced by laymen such as Dr. R. Cabot, Prof. William McDougall, and Dr. C. Macfie Campbell who were interested in mental health. Not suprisingly, Boisen prepared himself for a ministry to the mentally ill, and to train seminarians to become institutional chaplains. Before his illness Boisen had practiced his ministry in an interdenominational setting with secular co-workers familiar with the new techniques of the social sciences.[4]

On the invitation of Superintendent William A. Bryant, Boisen accepted a chaplaincy at Worcester State Hospital. He began his ministry by talking with the patients individually and then in groups.

In June of 1925 theological students began serving as attendants at Worcester State Hospital. They worked ten hours a day doing menial tasks. It was a hard and humble beginning for the first clinical training interns, and they had to battle for acceptance by the medical and psychiatric staffs.[5]

Outside funding was sought to permit work-study programs in place of working full time attendants. Students wanted to devote more time to what were traditionally considered to be ministerial duties such as writing letters for the patients, walking and talking with them and conducting recreational programs. Nevertheless seminarians kept careful case records of all their contacts with patients. Later they discussed their observations both with their theological supervisors and with the psychiatric staff of the hospital. Background information came from courses in psychiatry and religion and from attending staff meetings with Boisen and his psychiatric associates. But the lack of acceptance by other mental health workers remained a problem. The clinical training movement grew and clinical programs developed outside of mental hospitals. Student chaplains worked in general hospitals and prisons.

Financing the training programs was a chronic problem. Theological students who depended upon summer earnings to finance their studies during the regular school year could not afford to take part in a non-salaried summer training program. Their denominational organizations were unwilling to support interdenominational inter-disciplinary training institutes which they could not control. The cooperating institutions – usually prisons or mental institutions – lacked the funds to pay the clinical training interns.

Then, Philip Guiles, one of Boisen's early students, persuaded his father-in-law to donate money for this need. One stipulation which accompanied the gift was that Boisen and his followers would incorporate. This new body could be responsible for developing pro-grams for clinical training and for arranging for permanent funding.

The Council for Clinical Training for Theological Students was formed in January 21, 1930,[6] and Philip Guiles was its first executive secretary. The aim and hope of the movement was to make ministers into more effective pastoral counselors in their own parishes by providing opportunities to work with the more extreme forms of human suffereing often seen among institutionalized populations.[7] The Council was interdenominational, for it included Baptists, Episcopalians, and Congregationalists.

In 1934, the Federal Bureau of Prisons asked for Federal Council of Churches to nominate a candidate for the revised chaplaincy program. Wayne Hunter, a clinically trained minister who had been one of the first students in an experimental summer program in 1932, and had interned under Philip Guiles at the Massachusetts General Hospital, was the nominee of the Council. (The Federal Bureau of Prisons became the first body which supervised institutions to require inservice clinical training in addition to academic training for its chaplains.) In 1943, a full year training program in the Boston area was sponsored by the

Council for Clinical Training, in addition to several summer training institutes.

In 1932, the Council for Clinical Training moved to New York City. Fifteen years later it began to publish the *Journal of Pastoral Care.* The Council for Clinical Training now merged with the Institute for Pastoral Care, and with combined resources they sponsored programs for ministers and seminarians which emphasized growth through interpersonal relations. The basic philosophy of the institute was neo-Freudian.

By 1953 it had attracted fifty chaplain supervisors and over 200 ministers and seminarians as students. Twelve-week and full-term courses were offered in the techniques and limitations of counseling.[8]

The Institute for Pastoral Care had been organized in Boston in 1949 to facilitate better coordinated training programs. Most of the officers of the Institute were from seminaries located in the Boston area. However, Seward Hiltner, of Chicago, who was associated with the Federal Council of Churches, was active in the Institute, and lay workers in the field of mental health also served on the governing Board to insure that the quality of psychoanalytic training would be high.[9]

The Institute sought to expand the number of clinical training programs and insure that all training programs met certain minimum standards. At first two summer sessions were offered, one for seminarians and another for older experienced ministers. By 1953 the Institute was sponsoring nine summer institutes at different centers.

The focus of the clinical training movement quickly shifted from training chaplains for institutions to the larger market of training parish ministers. Clinical pastoral training was now urged for every minister.

Actually, The Institute for Pastoral Care could establish only limited control over the federated summer institutes. The Institute's requirements were that the supervising chaplains had to be clinically trained ministers who had received their training in hospitals or prisons. Resource people from the other mental health disciplines had to be available. The Institute reviewed conditions at the training facility annually and limited the number of enrollees. At the end of the summer session each student who successfully completed the course received a certificate from The Institute for Pastoral Care and a grade if his seminary required one.

Ernest Bruder established clinical pastoral training programs for ministers at St. Elizabeth's Hospital, a mental hospital for veterans in Washington, D. C., in cooperation with the Federal Council of Churches in Washington, D. C. The establishment of clinical training programs in veteran's hospitals was an outgrowth of the experience of the armed forces that clinical training of chaplains was necessary if the chaplains were to be effective in their pastoral work.

Bruder developed twelve-week courses of one whole or one half day per week for clergymen. Other goals of the program were to teach ministers about mental illness and enable them to continue pastoral care of the mentally ill of their congregation whether these were inside or outside of mental hospitals. The minister would also be able to detect early signs of mental illness and make appropriate and prompt referrals. Bruder also felt that training programs such as the one at St. Elizabeth's made churchmen more sensitive to signs of mental illness among other churchmen.

Ten to eighteen student chaplains who worked as interns at the hospital were supervised by Bruder. They were encouraged to live in the hospital for twelve weeks in order to familiarize themselves thoroughly with the problems of the mentally ill. Bruder was very concerned about the establishment of standards for clinical training programs. He required that all student chaplains possess a bachelor's degree and have completed their seminary studies. In addition, they were obligated to pass personal screening interviews. The course for ministers preparing to be institutional chaplains was a full year of internship after the completion of their collegiate and seminary studies. Those wishing to become training supervisors were required to serve another year of residency and to study psychology further.

During their residencies the chaplains attended staff conferences and lectures. Their chaplain supervisors held special seminars where the pastoral and religious concerns of the mental hospital ministry, mental illness, and the dynamics of personality were discussed. The duties of the student chaplains included conducting worship services and recreational activities. They had social contacts and religious interviews with the patients. Their studies were designed to enable them to complement and harmonize with the other members of the hospital mental health team.[10] A total of 150 clergymen participated in the training program at St. Elizabeth's Hospital between 1945 and 1955.[11]

In order to further the clinical training of pastoral counselors the Association for Clinical Pastoral Education was formed in 1957. The aim of the Association was to train ministers in the techniques of psychotherapy and thereby eventually enable the mentally ill to participate more fully in religious life.

In April 1963 a group of interested people established the American Association of Pastoral Counselors. The Association was composed of ministers who had received clinical training and were now working mainly in the parish ministry or in mental health centers throughout the nation. A year later the Association ratified a constitution, bylaws, and regulations drawn up by members of the Association during its first meeting. The initial concerns of the Association were standards for pastoral counselors and the establishment of different categories of membership corresponding to different skill levels.

Hiltner opposed the establishment of a hierarchy in the field of pastoral counseling. He preferred to concentrate on perfecting standards for clinical training programs and for the mental health centers in which many of the ministers worked. He pointed out that the Association was powerless to help the movement solve two of its most pressing problems, namely, financing of training programs and counseling centers, and denominational control of these centers.

It is likely that Hiltner was influenced by the sentiments of the deceased founder of the clinical training movement, Anton T. Boisen, who in 1948 had stated his opposition to any development such as the establishment of an association of pastoral counselors. Boisen felt that clinical training should be an integral part of every minister's seminary experience. He took pride in having trained 2,500 ministers by 1948. Boisen wrote, "I see neither the possibility nor the desirability of establishing a new profession of religious counselors."[12]

Hiltner, like Boisen, was more interested in providing a clinical training experience for all ministers rather than the establishment of a ministerial specialty. He said, "The model for pastoral counselors should be indigenous to them and to what if they are pastoral, they represent." In creating an association of pastoral counselors, one has the right to look for a specific education and training of a pastoral counselor.[13]

The debate over the proper role of the pastoral counselor continued. Howard J. Clinebell, when he was the head of the Association, tried to define the role of the pastoral counselor by saying that he was a specialist in pastoral counseling and should "have seminary training . . . be ordained and in good standing with his denomination . . . have advanced clinical and academic training in pastoral counseling and in one of the other counseling disciplines and hold the ministry as his primary professional identity." Clinebell, unlike Hiltner, felt that the Association would aid in "professional sharing and communication" standard setting, "interfaith cooperation," "interpretation," and "research."[14]

Clinebell was very aware of the difficulties involved in setting standards for this group. The standards had to be high enough to insure competence to handle the task at hand, and yet not so demanding as to render the group exclusive. There was the great danger that the new specialty of pastoral counselor might distort the traditional goals of the ministry. The pastoral counselor might de-emphasize the traditional ministerial functions and over-emphasize his specialty. In addition, the minister without specialized training might neglect his pastoral counseling duties because he felt less qualified than a fellow minister with clinical training experience.

Clinebell was also concerned about the development of pastoral counseling centers which functioned as community mental health centers. He relied upon the denominations involved to supervise the ministers who worked in these centers. Clearly this was not the most rigorous supervision. Only the most flagrant divergences from accepted attitudes and practices would come to the attention of the leaders of the denomination. The only punishment available to the leaders of the denomination would be removal from good standing, which was a very harsh punishment and rarely invoked. Another problem seen by Clinebell was that the ministers might adopt a particular type of counseling as a new orthodoxy, thus giving the pastoral counselors a unanimity that practicing psychologists and psychiatrists lacked. It seemed to Clinebell that the community mental health centers were the best way to extend the ministry of the clergy into the community. He hoped to improve pastoral counseling skills by having ministers participate in case conferences with other mental health workers. He advocated more advanced internships in pastoral counseling and institutes where ministers and laymen could study pastoral counseling together. Clinebell stressed that the unique function of the minister was to deal with the ontological anxiety of parishioners. Pastoral counseling centers outside of churches developed in the middle 1950s[15] and continued to grow in the 1960s, as the realization of the need for community health centers grew.[16]

Duane Parker, a minister who had worked at Topeka State Hospital, felt that religious resources were welcome at state hospitals. Medically trained people were no longer hostile towards religious workers in mental institutions. The contributions of pastoral counselors were now available and appreciated in community health centers.[17]

The clinical training movement had progressed greatly, a quarter century after its humble beginning in 1925. Clergymen and mental health workers were cooperating in mental health centers. Some of the leaders of the movement explained the reasons for its origin and continued growth. Clinical training enabled ministers to bring Christianity to the sick in hospitals and in other institutions.[18] Wayne E. Oates said that the minister had a role in the prevention of mental illness for which he needed the insights of psychology and sociology. Many mentally ill people experienced conflicts involving sexual behavior and loyalties,[19] and the minister could be of particular value in resolving these conflicts. Clinical training experience also helped ministers perform their regular pastoral duties more effectively.[20]

Ministers who participated in clinical training programs usually became enthusiastic supporters. They evaluated the program as having increased their self-awareness, helped in clarifying their roles as ministers and as religious teachers, and encouraged their personal growth as Christians.[21] In 1960, the clinical training movement had sufficiently matured to be able to study the effect of clinical training on seminarians.[22] Some of the changes included less authoritarian attitudes, a tendency towards conservative religious attitudes, and stronger religious feelings.

Another example of research and evaluation was the evaluation of Protestant Church pastoral counseling centers in 1961. This study found that pastoral counseling centers had developed from 1950 to 1960 mainly in urban centers; an eclectic but client-centered approach was used in therapy. They were well staffed by clerical and lay personnel. Most of the cases they saw involved marital difficulties. They received referrals from and made referrals to other agencies. They saw people who would not otherwise have received professional counseling. The authors felt that the Protestant counseling centers continued the tradition of seeing the neglected and helping them attain interpersonal and spiritual growth while avoiding more serious mental illness. The centers also provided ministers with opportunities for advanced training and expanded pastoral ministry.[23]

Some Catholic theologians thought that priests trained in psychology cooperating with Catholic psychiatrists and psychologists were needed to treat mentally ill Catholics. There were few calls for the clinical training of priests, and there was no discussion of curriculum of Catholic seminaries.[24]

Finlan McNamee described the clinical training program at St. Louis Hospital in St. Louis, Missouri in 1960. There were three levels of training. At the first level, newly ordained priests or seminarians in their last year of training attended lectures on psychology and mental illness and made pastoral visits to homes and to hospitals. This exposure to the theory and actuality of mental illness was designed to train priests to recognize its symptoms. Priests who wished to do special work with the mentally ill within the parish were enrolled in a program in which they spent twenty hours each week as counselor trainees in an institution and took university courses on related subjects. The third program was designed for those who wished to prepare themselves for a chaplain ministry. They were required to work as chaplain interns for one year and to take courses in related psychology and counseling.

There were several assumptions underlying the St. Louis program. In McNamee's words, divine grace could not be researched, today's mental health problems were insoluble, and mental health was not the ultimate Christian goal, although philosophy and science could help illuminate human behavior.[25]

Robert L. Katz described the beginnings of the clinical training at Hebrew Union College-Jewish Institute of Religion, the Reform Seminary in New York City where I. Fred Hollander formed the Jewish Council for Clinical Training on the Protestant model. There was no real parallel in Judaism to the Protestant clinical training movement. The practice of giving extensive pastoral care did not exist in Judaism. Hollander served as the clinically trained supervisor for five rabbinical students who participated in a clinical training program. The movement was based upon the philosophy of Joshua Loth Liebman who stressed the importance of love, self-acceptance, and good interpersonal relations.[26]

In 1957, the Jewish Theological Seminary of America, a Conservative seminary, established a Department of Psychiatry. Jewish doctors of medicine taught principles of psychiatry to rabbinical students. A Jewish literature of pastoral psychology had not been developed. The articles which existed were published in *Pastoral Psychology*, a Protestant journal. Simon Noveck referred rabbis to *Pastoral Psychology* for advice on the application of psychology to religion, telling the rabbis that they should ignore the explicit Christian references.[27] Reform and Conservative theological seminaries taught clinical psychology accompanied by some case studies, rather than pastoral psychology. They offered little or no clinical training. Rabbis desiring a master's degree in counseling took courses at the Institute for Pastoral Care in New York City.

By 1965 a new group of mainly Protestant professionals had emerged; they drew from the field of psychology and religion to create a pastoral psychology. They trained seminarians and ordained ministers in this new discipline, and they tried to professionalize the pastoral counselors by developing standards for accreditation of individuals and training programs. The goal of pastoral psychologists was to make the minister more effective as he executed his pastoral duties. Pastoral visits to the sick and to the well, in private homes, institutions, or at counseling centers were to be based upon a pastoral theology which was psychologically valid. Throughout the development of the clinical training movement, the liberal Protestant denominations provided the leadership and organized the interdenominational organizations, like the

Institute for Pastoral Care, through which ministers of all faiths often obtained clinical pastoral training.

The Role of Ministers and Institutional Chaplains

In the post–World War II era, ministers were uncertain of their new role as pastoral counselors. Changed patterns of living and working, where often both members of the family were employed, made the old style of pastoral visitation difficult. In its place many ministers assumed a mental health role, utilizing the time which was formerly spent visiting congregants for therapeutic sessions at the church, the mental health center, or even at the counselee's home. Ministers and psychologists explored the areas of ministerial competence. They also discussed the problem of reconciling religious morality with the non-judgmental attitudes required for the success of counseling. Ministers assimilated as much of the technique and philosophy of counseling as they felt was compatible with their ministerial roles.

Clergymen began to feel that they had a responsibility for and an interest in the mental health of the community. They studied psychology to learn about the emotional life of the individual and tried to emphasize by deed and by teaching concepts of proper adult behavior.[28] Ministers thought that they should also be familiar with community mental health agencies in order to work with them or make referrals to them.[29] After World War II there was much more interest in the role of the minister as a mental health counselor, since an increasing number of ministers were trained in psychology and were also more aware of mental health problems.

William Menninger, a psychiatrist well known to the general public, discussed the kinds of therapy a minister was capable of doing. The pastor should practice both supportive and preventive therapy. He noted, however, that ministers rarely had the training for depth therapy.[30] In answer to the question of how far a minister should progress in therapy with an extreme neurotic, Menninger had concluded by 1952 that he should continue until neurotic symptoms of a physical nature appeared, in which case medical help was necessary. In another answer to this question, Russell Baker, a pastoral psychologist, said that the minister should continue as long as he felt comfortable in the therapeutic situation. On the other hand, Carroll Wise, also a pastoral psychologist, insisted that the average minister had neither the time nor the training to treat an extreme neurotic.[31]

Charles F. Brooks, a minister, addressed himself to the same problem in 1951. Pastoral counseling, he declared, had to be limited by the teachings of Jesus Christ and the Gospels and by belief in God and immortality. He felt that few pastors had the training to conduct depth therapy, although many were effective in marriage counseling.[32] Thomas Bingham added in 1952 that a pastor was a judge, a teacher, a father, and a physician of souls. In his counseling he should emphasize the positive nature of sexual experience and the sacred and solid nature of marriage.[33] Anton T. Boisen underlined the role of prayer in counseling. No minister should forget that prayer could be of special help in allowing people to share their worries and obtain relief from irrational and obsessive symptoms.[34]

Meanwhile, Karl Menninger in 1958 discussed the difficult problem of accepting the client while rejecting some of his actions which contravened Christian morality. He advised that the minister acting as a pastoral psychologist should make a moral judgment on a client's future plans but avoid condemning a client's past actions. The pastor should also resist the temptation to shape the patient in the pastor's image.[35]

The pastor was a perpetual therapist who tried to improve the interpersonal relations of his parishioners at work, at play, at church, and with their families and thereby increase their enjoyment of life, said John Sutherland Bonnell. Therefore, he should be as skilled as possible in techniques of counseling.[36] In 1965, A. Mansell Pattison further explored the multifaceted role of the clergyman as a mental health counselor. He suggested that the counselor functioned as a religious counselor, as a diagnostician, as a general mental health worker, and as a consultant who was attuned to the voice of the community.[37]

Wayne E. Oates focused upon techniques of counseling for ministers. First he stressed the importance of creative listening, creative because people could then express themselves through their bodies. Silences could be very provocative. Oates believed that the therapist should try to encourage the patient to talk, although he shied away from non-directive therapy which he identified as the method of Carl Rogers.[38] The steps in the therapeutic process, said Oates, were gaining of insight, remembering repressed material, and admission of "ambivalent" feelings.[39]

But Seward Hiltner reminded readers that acceptance of negative feelings and understanding the cause of rebellion were also important.[40] He maintained that pastoral counseling was decidedly different from psychotherapy. The church setting itself accounted for some of the difference. Supportive therapy was the technique, and the ultimate aim of counseling was salvation and redemption, although there might be other goals. The counseling relationship complicated other relationships within the church. When counseling took place on neutral ground, the

Christian nature of the counseling was lessened and therapy took on a more neutral tone.[41]

Glenn V. Ramsey listed warning signs of emotional disorders which required treatment. Chief of these were hyperactivity and lethargy, psychosomatic illness, odd behavior, tension-reducing habits, periods of unconsciousness, negative self-image, rebelliousness, anxiety, and sleep or speech disorders.[42]

The Catholic conception of the role of the priest changed less than had been the case with Protestants. Although the priest brought God's love and forgiveness to the penitent, he remained primarily the upholder of moral law and a directive counselor. The insights of psychology had very little impact on this role. Possibly in institutional chaplaincies the priest functioned more like his Protestant counterpart, offering love, fellowship, and forgiveness and concerning himself with breaches in moral law only when he felt that the patient was ready to consider his sin. In the parish ministry, however, the influence of psychology on Catholicism and on American culture in general meant that the priest would be more likely to recognize signs of mental illness such as scrupulosity and obsessional confessions, and refer the penitent or parishioner to the appropriate mental health worker. Ideally, there would be a psychologist-priest, or a priest with some clinical training available to treat mental health problems. If not, a referral might be made to a Catholic social service organization or practitioner who perferably was a practicing Catholic or at least a religious person. The ability to identify a mental health problem and distinguish it from a religious problem was a step forward.

Rudolph Allers defined the role of the priest in psychological terms. He said that the priest had to try to help the penitent control his "irresistible impulses." While a psychiatrist or a psychologist might acknowledge that the penitent in his role as a patient might have irresistible impulses, the priest had to continue to help the penitent to control them.[43] Charles A. Currian thought that the pastoral counselor had to be aware of the workings of God in every person.[44]

Odenwald and VanderVeldt concluded that the role of the priest in mental health was that of a empathetic counselor and confessor. As a confessor he had to assess penance for all the conscious sins committed by the penitent. When there was illness in the family, either mental or physical, his pastoral visits would influence the home environment and help maintain sound family life. Obviously the priest should have knowledge of mental illness in order to make referrals to competent psychiatrists or psychologists. The average priest should not attempt to practice psychotherapy because he was not qualified to do so. Therefore, it would be advantageous to have priests who were trained as psychotherapists in the diocese. In general the priest and the psychiatrist should cooperate, although they had different spheres.[45]

Currian added that the priest and the psychotherapist had in common that they both related to the client in a spirit of love, acceptance, and optimism. The theological needs of man were another dimension which existed outside of the realm of the psychiatrist.

The role of the rabbi was quite different from that of a Protestant minister. Traditionally rabbis did little or no pastoral work which could be compared to the pastoral visitation and counseling done by Protestant ministers. Although a person might ask the rabbi for advice, the existence of Jewish social and welfare organizations outside of and apart from the synagogue made it unlikely that the rabbi would do more than refer the person to an appropriate agency.

The different branches of Judaism reacted differently to psychology, depending upon their outlook toward the world. In the most traditional branches, such as Orthodox and Hasidic Judaism, the rabbi spent much of his day in leading group prayer and studying traditional religious books. He would most likely know little or nothing of modern psychology and see very little reason to concern himself with it. He would have enough knowledge to refer congregants to appropriate mental health agencies and would probably do so. In addition, he might offer prayers for the individual's recovery during the group worship service. For an Orthodox Jew, the aim of life was the fulfillment of God's commandments, not the attainment of mental health.

In the middle branch of American Judaism, Conservative Judaism, the rabbi would have more knowledge of the secular world than would the Orthodox rabbi. His main job would be running the synagogue which was a community center.[46]

Freudian and neo-Freudian psychology had their greatest impact on Reform Judaism, because the Reform branch was the most influenced by American culture and the least involved in ritual observances. The Reform rabbi had more time to develop his role as a counselor.

The role of the rabbi differed from that of the Protestant minister or the Catholic priest. The rabbi was a teacher, a group leader, a preacher, a mentor, a public figure, an advocate of the Jews among the Christians, and also a counselor and a therapist.[47] Even a rabbi with a great interest in counseling could only spend a very limited amount of time counseling without seriously neglecting his other duties, which in the eyes of most Jews would have precedence.

I. Fred Hollander investigated the role of the rabbi in promoting mental health in a study conducted in cooperation with Yeshiva

University in New York City, with funds provided by the National Institute of Health.[48]   Hollander said that the clergy could encourage mental health by outlining a program of healthful living.   They should have an awareness of signs of mental illness in order to begin treatment early or make prompt referrals.   Clergymen should learn from other disciplines the information and techniques necessary to understand and to help treat mental illness.   In addition, the traditional resources of religion could be brought to bear on mental health.   The customs, ethics and morality of religion could be used to encourage mental health. Religion offered opportunities for self-fulfillment and for communication with others.   Hollander also advocated clinical training for rabbis because he thought that it would enable rabbis to deal more effectively with the mentally ill and with normal people.[49]

Enoch Kagan, a rabbi who accepted existential philosophy, argued in 1954 that that rabbi should function as a pastoral psychologist, administering projective psychological tests even if he had to ask the aid of a clinical psychologist in interpreting them.   The rabbi should also be a good listener and offer acceptance to those who came to him for advice.   By functioning as a permissive pastoral counselor, Kagan said that that the rabbi could give people the "courage to be."[50]

Although Kagan believed that all of the rabbi's contacts with people should be therapeutic,[51] most rabbis preferred a more traditional role and left testing to the psychologists.   There were great differences between the role of the rabbi and the role of the psychotherapist.   The rabbi could be trained in counseling, but he could not be non-judgmental; in this respect there was a profound difference between the rabbi and the psychotherapist.   When someone was violating God's law the rabbi had to take a moral position on evil and possibly rebuke him. The rabbi's value sytem was based upon revelation which was based in turn upon tradition.   Moreover, the rabbi was not trained to handle the specific problems of a therapeutic relationship, such as the problems of transference and countertransference.   The rabbi could, however, give comfort.[52]

Enoch Kagan set a high goal for the rabbi when he said that the door to his home was always open and that he was applying therapy in all his interpersonal relationships.   This attitude suggests the extent to which attitudes favorable to psychotherapy had permeated liberal American culture by the 1960s.

The role of the rabbi as conceived by American Jews was different from and more complex than that of the Protestant minister.   The rabbi was the foremost spiritual leader of the Jewish community, and also the final moral arbiter.   Most American rabbis devoted much of their time and attention to a religious school which functioned afternoons, evenings and weekends, and to other communal activities.   In addition, rabbis considered that they had the role of interpreter of the Jewish community to the Christian world.   Most rabbis felt that they had little time to assume new counseling duties.[54]

Protestant ministers seemed to be involved in psychotherapy more than were priests and rabbis.   They therefore debated the role of the minister as a counselor more extensively.   They concluded that the minister might proceed with therapy to the extent that he felt competent, at whatever location the therapy took place.   When he no longer felt competent or able to devote sufficient time to a counselee, he should make a referral to another mental health professional.   Priests and rabbis followed similar guidelines, although they generally had less clinical pastoral traning, devoted less time to counseling, and would generally be more likely to refer a congregant requiring therapy to another mental health professional.   Priests also expressed concern about the moral consequence of non-directive therapy.   Ministers of all faiths were concerned that their counseling be psychologically valid and religiously oriented at the same time.   They decided that their aim of bringing a counselee closer to God could best be achieved through non-directive methods of counseling, which they called client-centered therapy.   In general, they felt that they could not avoid but they could delay making moral judgments.

Chaplains in institutions, and in mental hospitals in particular, were constantly dealing with individuals experiencing emotional crises.   They were among the first to call for the clinical training of institutional chaplains, because they realized that traditional Protestant pastoral theology did not contain the methodology or insight that was necessary in order to alleviate the sufferings of people in institutions.   The first clinically trained ministers served as chaplains in mental hospitals, and later in general hospitals, and prisons long before clinical pastoral training was usually part of the preparation of a parish minister.   The twin problems of Protestant hospital chaplaincy programs were financing and recognition of the specialized ministry as a profession.

Don C. Shaw surveyed the duties of a chaplain in a state hospital in 1947.   He said that a chaplain should conduct Sunday worship services, counsel patients in emergencies, and work with all patients. Both new patients and patients already under treatment needed the personal attention of the minister.   He could provide patients with suitable reading material, and should cooperate with the rest of the hospital staff.   The minister had to be capable of orderly thinking if he were to exercise insight into the problems of the patients.   In addition, he had to offer acceptance and fellowship. If he met these criteria, religion would be a healing agent.[55]

In 1947, Ernest Bruder asserted that a clinically trained chaplain could be very supportive of patients in a mental hospital. Through the use of worship services the minister could overcome the isolation of the patient and help him to begin to form relationships within the hospital community.[56]

The function of the worship service in a mental hospital also had the support of Anton Boisen. For instance, the chaplain should exercise special care in his choice of hymns; these should stress forgiveness of sins and man's aspirations, and celebrate special occasions. The aim of the worship service would be to integrate the individual into the community, and for that purpose the group should cultivate a family-like atmosphere.[57]

In 1949, chaplains recognized the importance of love, as the basis of the relationship between the chaplain and patients. Religious faith was dependent upon love. Authoritarian attitudes which stemmed from fear led to distorted religious beliefs. The most important quality a chaplain needed to possess was all-encompassing love.[58]

Russell C. Dicks, a leader in the clinical training movement, stressed the importance of love in a chaplain's relationship with his patients. He held that preaching was not needed, but a warm accepting relationship in which the chaplain could be a living example of God's love was essential. Dicks said that as of 1940 only 11 out of 518 Protestant hospitals possessed ordained Protestant chaplains. Catholic chaplains, on the other hand, were found much more commonly in hospitals. The reason for the sparsity of Protestant institutional chaplains was that few Protestant institutions were willing to finance chaplaincy programs. After World War II, veteran's hospitals were served by Protestant chaplains who were paid by the government of the United States. He noted that state hospitals and non-sectarian private hospitals were constrained from hiring chaplains and the salaries had to come from private sources. Dicks suggested that rich churches or local councils of churches finance chaplaincy programs in their communities and that hospital chaplains be recognized as specialized professionals. A hopeful sign in the development of a specialized institutional ministry was that seminaries were now hiring institutional chaplains to teach courses in pastoral counseling.[59] The report in 1954 that the chaplain at an Illinois boys' training school was really working as a psychotherapist[60] probably reflects only the way that the adminstration of the school was able to justify paying the chaplain's salary.

Calvin Hall discussed the objectives of a psychiatric chaplain who worked with religious literature. Personally, he tried to achieve inter-action among group members while accepting any interpretation of the story. He also tried to help the patients identify with the characters in the stories and work out some of their personal problems through that identification.[61]

There was no discussion of the role of the Catholic institutional chaplain in the relevant literature, but Catholic chaplains probably func-tioned much like their Protestant counterparts.

There were few full time Jewish chaplains in institutions because of the small number of Jews in institutions. Most Jewish chaplains served on a part-time and most often on a volunteer basis. They encountered the same problems as did their Protestant counterparts. I. M. Melamed said that the Jewish prisoners he encountered had suffered from a lack of love as children and a lack of discipline in the home.[62]

Ministry to Special Groups

Pastoral counselors realized that groups such as alcoholics and their families, the retarded, the divorced, delinquent children, and homosexuals required that the general principles of neo-Freudian pastoral counseling be applied in ways which would create a feeling of love and acceptance of the counselee by the counselor, thereby establishing good object relations. Pastoral psychologists and other mental health workers contributed articles detailing the problems involved in working with these special groups and suggesting techniques or making observations which grew out of their experience.

Pastoral counselors realized that special problems required special skills and presented special difficulties. Robert V. Seliger noted that an alcoholic who experienced a true religious or conversion experience would be able to redirect his life. He would be less self-centered and more interested in others, and he might achieve peace of mind.[63] Religious counseling should be directed towards achieving this orientation.

Howard J. Clinebell was a leader in the clinical training movement. He considered that an alcoholic was a sick person in need of help rather than a sinner as depicted in much past theological litereature and in many sermons.[64] Joan K. Jackson said that families of alcoholics should be helped to realize that alcoholism was a sickness and not evidence of sinfulness. A minister could help them by offering sustaining faith in God.[65] E. A. Verdery said that pastoral care of the alcoholic and his family had to continue after his reintroduction into the community.[66] Clinebell suggested that when counseling an alcoholic's family before the alcoholic achieved sobriety, the pastoral counselor should reintroduce them to the community, and give them help with acute problems and information about alcoholism. The minister should explain to the family that the alcoholic must hit bottom and surrender before there could be a real change in his behavior. The wife should be led to examine whether she had any neurotic tendencies which encouraged her husband to be weak and dependent.[67]

The special problem that the homosexual presented to the pastoral counselor was discussed by Alfred A. Gross in 1950. Gross recommended that the minister should help the homosexual who came for help by trying to relieve his guilt feelings about his homosexuality, and then guide him to accept himself and regain his self-respect. Possibly the minister should also make a referral to a therapist.[68]

Aaron L. Rutledge said that people with personality problems tended to identify with God in different ways although the most universal presumption was that God cared for them. Hymns encouraged different kinds of identification. Some hymns fostered homosexual or heterosexual identification and many pictures of Jesus depicted him as having a somewhat effeminate appearance. The minister could choose the most appropriate material for the group with which he was working.[69] However, Edmund Bergler said that he treated homosexuality as a masochistic neurotic disorder.[70]

Hubert Hendin discussed ministering to another group, potential suicides. He warned that the minister had to know when to intervene to prevent a suicide, at a time when a dependent person lost the protector upon whom his security was based. Lovers' quarrels represented another but less serious threat to life.[71]

F. C. Cesarman described his personal technique with a male sex offender. Using neo-Freudian psychology, Cesarman said that he first made the offender aware of the relationship between the offender and the observer. Then the therapist put himself in the place of the observer and ultimately the patient was able to tolerate a strong relationship between himself and the church which gave him enough security that he was able to stop his exhibitionist behavior.[72]

In 1953, Judson D. Howard showed a sophisticated understanding of the role the minister could play in aiding the recovery of a hospitalized mental patient. Giving the hospitalized mental patient normal pastoral care would aid his reentry into normal society. A supportive religious counselor might help the patient recover because improved interpersonal relations were often the key element in a patient's recovery. Supportive therapy by the minister could sometimes avoid the necessity of hospitalization. Howard showed familiarity with neo-

Freudian psychology and with the newest ideas about the hospitalization of the mentally ill.[73]

John Sutherland Bonnell discussd the divorced as a special category of counseling. First, it was important to make the client understand the neurotic pattern which caused the divorce, in order to prevent a recurrence of the pattern.[74]   Charles William Stewart added that in counseling divorcees the emphasis should be on helping people accept the changes in their life wrought by the divorce and to accept the responsibility for the changes.[75]

The retarded needed a special ministry. A minister to the retarded first had to work through any feelings of revulsion he might have towards retarded people. The ministry to the retarded should include helping parents to accept their child's retardation. Short simple church services for the retarded could aid in improving interpersonal relations in the homes for the retarded.[76]

Pastoral ministry to children was probably the most important special ministry and the first to develop. The turmoil of World War II and of the postwar era placed great strains on family life, resulting in increased restlessness and delinquency among youth.

Milton I. Levine and Reuel L. Howe stressed the importance of security and parent-child affection during the first six years of the child's life. It was during this time that the child learned to receive love, which enabled him to manage his hostilities.[77]   Anna Freud wrote of the need for good object relations for the development of the child and the management of hostility after caring for English children who were separated from their parents as a result of World War II.   Stuart McIntyre Finch said in 1951 that the anxious child was afraid of his inner urges and that the minister should interfere in the family situation with gentle suggestions. The child had to be taught to understand his emotions, and defenses against them should not be developed.[78]   Finch accepted the Freudian definition of anxiety as the result of the suppression of the libido by the ego. Samuel Southard noted that the parent's relationship with the child was of key importance in determining the attitude of the child in joining the church.[79]

In 1956, Earl Loomis pointed out that child psychiatry and religion had common goals in the well-being of the child. Both recognized the importance of the early stages of development in determining future attitudes.   Loomis said that the core or the balance in the child's personality was the ego. At first the child depended upon the mother's ego, but eventually he developed his own. The relationship between the mother and the child had to be a balance between naturalness and spontaneity combined with at least some firm guidelines on behavior.

The mother had to practice what she taught in order for her teaching to be effective.[80]

In the postwar period ministers had to counsel children whose parents were divorced. Divorce presented children with difficult problems to which they often reacted by experiencing rage, hate, or pity. When parents asked children to take sides in parental disagreements, the emotional conflicts of the children intensified. Divorce situations presented fewer problems to the children when the children were given adequate explanations of what happened.[81] John H. Snow stressed the importance of knowing when it was necessary to refer "troublesome" children to other agencies.[82]

Techniques of Counseling

Pastors embarking on the new field of psychologically-oriented pastoral counseling tried to develop a philosophy of counseling which would be a combination of psychoanalytic insights and Christian philosophy.

Earl Ferguson in 1948 noted the importance of accepting the patient as he was. He advocated the use of preaching to show the minister as a sympathetic human being who could establish ethical and moral standards for the community upon which the therapeutic relationship could be based. Thus, the client would know what was expected in terms of ethical behavior before the counseling began.[83] In 1941, Seward Hiltner had expressed a similar concern that normative behavior be established before the counseling relationship was begun in order to properly define the relationship. Hiltner believed that dynamic psychology had to be employed, while professional therapeutic standards were met by the keeping of case records, preaching, reflection, and understanding on the part of the counselor.[84]

Client-centered therapy in a Christian context was advocated by Ralph Higgins as the philosophical framework for therapy in 1949. He advocated the use of Gestalt psychology in the larger context of embracing the entire world including the divine instead of the secular world only. The minister should emphasize unifying the entire personality in order to enable the parishioner to grow, end his suffering and restore his trust in man and in God. Higgins said that client-centered therapy was applicable both to the sick and the well.

Client-centered therapy put the will in its proper place because its eventual success enabled the person to make his own decisions and practice free will. The pastor had to deal with man's sinful state by speaking in terms of original sin without ever losing his non-judgmental attitude toward the client. The ultimate aim of therapy was salvation, which meant reconciliation with God. Higgins saw a potential problem in the counseling situation when the minister's concern for the patient's immediate happiness conflicted with his concern for the parishioner's salvation.[85]   Wayne E. Oates noted that religious fellowship groups, counseling, and worship services could all be used by the minister to re-socialize psychotic mental patients.[86]

Russell C. Dicks in 1951 reflected upon types of questions which might be employed by the pastor, and techniques of discussion. According to Harry Stack Sullivan, said Dicks, direct questioning was doomed to failure; pressing to the heart of the matter too fast was a form of aggression.   Dicks listed different types of questions including those designed to cause reflection on the part of the parishioner and those which elicited information which the minister needed to know.[87]

Howard Clinebell gave attention to techniques of counseling in 1963.   He found the key concepts of pastoral counseling theory in the theory of unconscious motivation, the childhood roots of behavior, the development of insight as the goal of counseling process, and the utilization of a non-directive client-centered method.   The crucial element in counseling was the relationship between counselor and counselee. There were various types of supportive therapy, including crisis-oriented therapy and sustaining therapy.[88]

Catholics thought that priests had to remain directive counselors, because they could not be non-directive and uphold the teachings of the Church.   A. B. Bioren charged that Rogerian therapy, which was permissive and non-directive, conflicted with Catholic doctrine by denying the objective nature of truth.[89]   Most Catholic pastoral counselors still believed that in order to uphold moral law they were required to practice directive counseling.

Odenwald and VanderVeldt expressed a similar preference for directive over non-directive counseling.   They emphasized that every Catholic counselor had to adhere to the teachings of the Church and make clear to the patient when his behavior violated moral law. However, they recognized that there were times when the patient could not control his impulse to sin and when he was not ready to listen to appropriate counsel.[90]

Charles A. Currian said in 1958 that the relationship of the client to the counselor paralleled man's relationship to God, but the counselor had to go beyond Freudian psychology to Augustinian philosophy in order to give meaning to the client's life.[91]   William C. Bier distinguished between guidance, counseling, and psychotherapy in 1959.   Guidance was derived from education and had the education of the client as its primary aim.

Counseling, on the other hand, was derived from psychotherapy which was concerned with disorders. The aim of counseling was to make the client think through his problems in order to find good solutions. Counseling was also concerned with attitudes rather than actions and with relationships with other people.

It was only in the decade of the 1950s, said Bier, that clergymen came to think of themselves as counselors and to assume a counseling rather than a guidance role. One reason for the change was that many clergymen found that mere sympathy and advice were not effective in changing parishioner behavior or helping parishioners solve their problems. However, clergymen remained religious counselors with the ultimate aim of bringing the client closer to God and to salvation. Counseling was only one of their pastoral functions, and not the principal one either. Religious counseling also aimed at helping the client achieve a more conflict-free and less inhibited religious life, in which the client would feel it easier to accept God's plan. Bier cautioned that serious personality disorders should be referred to a psychotherapist.[92] Peter F. Girende and Nathaniel J. Paollome wondered to what extent the religious role of the therapist inhibited psychotherapy.[93]

Existentialism had a relatively slight influence on Judaism. In 1956, Harry J. Brevis said that he used the Rogerian technique of reflecting back to the client what he said in the course of therapy. By doing so he helped to create new self-awareness among prisoners.[94]

Jewish writers were less concerned with techniques of counseling than Protestant or Catholic theologians, probably because they did less counseling. They wrote of the importance of acceptance of the client by the counselor, but in most cases the rabbi probably functioned in a very directive manner. One study indicates that rabbis were not good listeners.[95]

Group therapy was a major innovation in mental health treatment in the 1950s. Clinical pastoral counselors tried group counseling as did many other mental health workers. Ministers perceived many advantages in group therapy. The therapeutic group was seen as an extension of the traditional Christian fellowship group. Group therapy was more economical; the cost to the individual patient was less, while the minister could see more patients. Pastors felt that they were making better use of the time devoted to counseling. There was less resistance to group than to individual therapy because fellowship groups had traditionally been used to strengthen relationships within the Christian community. The moral stigma traditionally associated with mental illness could be hidden. The therapeutic group resembled the traditional fellowship group, bringing together lonely people who were seeking to broaden and enrich their lives. The group could also provide information to the minister about the needs for expanded church activities.

In 1951, the Rev. Robert Leslie, a leading advocate of group therapy, said that it should become part of the clinical pastoral training program. He explained the dynamic process of group therapy; "the goal of group discussions is always to uncover the deeper more personal dynamic implications of the subject."   Leslie described the progress of a therapeutic group as beginning with the "testing out" process of the libido followed by a period of "resistance" during which time the patients exhibited hostility to the non-directive methods of group counseling. The more postive phase followed (which he called the "acceptance" phase) when the group worked out problems and showed "responsibility" for its direction and itself.[96]

In 1955, the Revs. Clifton E. and Clinton J. Kew, both advocates of group therapy as a type of pastoral counseling, wrote about the problems caused by resistance and by transference in group counseling. They attributed resisitance to "first unconscious drives, impulses, repressed associations and traumatic experiences and, second to transference and counter-transference." They defined transference as the "unconscious emotional displacement of feeling and emotions from another situation to the therapeutic one."[97]

To the Kews, group therapy offered many advantages. They felt that more varied transference took place more rapidly in a group situation. The group could be supportive of individuals. They felt that "the patients strengthened their egos by assuming roles of responsibility towards one another." They also said that "attitudes and feelings related to the original family are brought out and the patient is able to see his neurotic behavior in action, and the relation of his behavior to his childhood past."   In fact, the group could function as a substitute and better family for the members. The permissive atmosphere and common goals of the new family established a rapport and reduced fear and guilt.

In 1951, Clifton E. Kew described some of the mechanics of group therapy. Certainly, a patient had to be prepared for his entry into the therapeutic group.   The therapist had to gather biographical data, determine the individual's personality structure and his problems. The structure and dynamics of group therapy, and the phenomena of transference, free association, the functions of dreams and fantasies, and the meaning of working through one's problem had to be explained. The role of the clergyman was that of bringing forth the irrational frustrations, anxiety and hostility within the group members to enable them to experience peace, relaxation, and the ability to love.[98]

Rollin J. Fairbanks advocated the formation of preventive therapy groups within the church in 1951.[99]   C. W. Hyde and R. C. Leslie suggested that graduate theological students might work with disturbed adults and with peer groups to become aware of the kinds of personal growth that could be fostered in adults when ministers refrained from assuming authoritarian attitudes.[100]   Anton T. Boisen wrote supportively about holding group therapy discussions in the convalescent and admission wards of Elgin State Hospital where he used music at therapy sessions.   Boisen emphasized facing moral problems and difficulties honestly; thus he gave therapy a Christian context.[101]   Clifton E. Kew asserted that confession in group therapy was like free association because the confessing was done in an atmosphere of love. He felt that there was less strain on the client's ego than during individual private confessions and with less disturbance due to aggression.[102]

Ministers found many advantages in group therapy.   By receiving therapy in fellowship groups the patient escaped the stigma of being mentally ill.   Also some patients exhibited less resistance and found it easier to expose their feelings earlier in a group than in individual therapy.   Although certain emotions were easily expressed to the individual therapist, there could be more varied transference within the group.   In addition, the group provided real life situations in which patients could test their emotional reactions within the group and develop better interpersonal relations.   In a group situation, "attitudes and feelings" which related to childhood situations were quickly exposed, and the patient was able to see how his neurotic behavior was related to his childhood and how it affected others. The group could examine the meaning of dreams together.   They could serve as a permissive loving and accepting new family which would reduce fear and guilt among the group members.

Robert C. Leslie sketched the history of group therapy in 1955. It began in the army with non-medical leadership.   The purpose of the groups was to alleviate psychoneuroses.   Certain conditions had to be met for therapy groups to be successful.   The aims of the group had to be clearly stated.   Fellowship was not a substitute for self-inquiry which was essential for the progress of therapy.   Members had to show concern for the feelings of other group members.   There had to be attention given to current activities, to intergroup relations between members, and between members and the leader.   The role of the leader and the way that it differed from the usual authoritarian style of the group leader had to be understood.   Sessions should last one and one-half hours, and the leader should keep case records detailing the progress of the group.[103]

Leslie believed that adjustment to the group preceded adjustment to the world.[104]   Russell Dicks thought that laymen could be trained in "nurture groups" to do pastoral visiting.[105] Others searched the Bible and found evidence of group dynamics and group interaction. Groups could be used for therapy and for study.[106] Religious psychodrama could be employed to focus the attention of the group on religious programs.[107] Others praised group pastoral counseling because it was more economical in terms of the use of the minister's time. Group therapy also had the advantages of providing company for people who might be lonely, and making the minister aware of the problems of the parishioners, which might otherwise escape his notice. The minister could then try to satisfy some of those needs by establishing new activities and addressing his preaching to those needs.[108]

Thus, group counseling provided a low cost, socially acceptable method of counseling more parishioners than the minister could otherwise reach.

Validation of the "Call to the Ministry"

Protestant theologians had to differentiate a valid "call to the ministry" from cases of psychopathology. One way of differentiating was to use projective psychological tests in seminaries to try to exclude those who were deemed psychologically unfit. Although the veracity of a "call" was never denied, only well-integrated individuals were considered to be suitable candidates for the seminary. In 1949, the Episcopal Church began requiring that candidates for ordination to the ministry pass a psychiatric examination.[109]

Protestant writers realized that ordination did not guarantee mental health. Roy Burkhart, for example, conceded that a minister might need psychiatric help to free himself of neurotic conflicts.[110]

Blanche Carrier discussed the psychological problems she had encountered in counseling candidates for the seminary. She noted that many had come with problems which resulted from repressed anxieties often caused by the withdrawal of love. Sometimes withdrawal of love did not result in anxiety, but was manifested as defiance, withdrawal, or castigation. Pre-ministerial students occasionally suffered from guilt, but usually they were able to release guilt through a conversion experience. Sometimes guilt was not released but was displaced and resulted in warping of the entire personality. Carrier said that counseling was often helpful in releasing a patient from a neurotic image of God, but at times failed to build another healthy substitute image, and the individual was left without faith.[111]

Some seminaries employed psychiatrists as consultants. C. W. Christensen discussed the role of the psychiatric consultant. The psychiatrist could examine candidates for the ministry and discuss their motivations with them. He could encourage candidates to undergo psychotherapy when he thought that therapy was needed. He could also teach techniques of counseling to seminarians and to the ministers of the community for whom he could also be a resource for those who needed psychiatric treatment. The psychiatrist could also function as a therapist for the faculty of the seminary.[112]

Daniel Blain thought that seminarians should receive psychotherapy in order to rid themselves of neurotic compulsions which arose in the unconscious while they were preparing for the ministry. Seminarians should also be prepared for difficulties commonly present in a ministerial career, such as poverty and the need to repress the expression of normal emotions, to be self-sacrificing, and to endure the pressure towards conformity.[113] M. O. Williams said that psychological evaluation should be part of the selection process for missionaries as well. The process should include the use of psychiatric interviews.[114]

Verifying a ministerial "call" also concerned Carroll Wise. He felt that a call to the ministry could be understood by one who was psychologically oriented in terms of his emotional and intellectual life and his attitude towards himself and others. Wise noted that psychological observations of a person would reveal the person's inner dynamics but could not validate a ministerial call. Similarly, he found projective tests to be a useful diagnostic tool but of no therapeutic value.[115]

Others recognized the problem. Margaretta K. Bowers said that a theologically healthy person was one in whom theological and psychological truths coincided. She felt that man had to experience human love before he could experience God's love.[116] H. B. Schoelfield, a minister who underwent psychoanalysis, said that as the result of analysis he realized that his unconscious conflicts had interfered with his sermonizing. He thought that ministers who did pastoral counseling brought new life to the parishioners.[117]

By the 1950s Catholic seminaries were testing seminarians with projective psychological tests and psychiatric interviews. There was no discussion in the relevant literature of criteria for verifying a ministerial call, nor was there any discussion of the psychological problems of priests, although the problems of nuns did receive some attention.

During the same decade psychology courses were being offered at the Reform and Conservative rabbinical seminaries. By the 1960s some Orthodox seminaries were listing courses in psychology. Most Orthodox and Hasidic rabbis probably had no knowledge of psychology.[118]

Abraham Franzblau, who taught psychology courses at the Hebrew Union College–Jewish Institute of Religion in New York City, advocated that all candidates for the rabbinate undergo a psychological examiniation before ordination, but there is no indication that his recommendation was ever put into effect.

Ministers of all faiths were aware of psychosomatic illness. Its existence was often cited to demonstrate the wholeness of man which was postulated in most religious philosophies. Ministers were willing to work with the medical and psychological professions to help alleviate psychosomatic suffering.

Gothard Booth said in 1951 that religion and psychiatry could work together to cure psychosomatic illness. He thought that a reorientation of the personality could occur through a conversion experience, with the attendant surrender and loss of pride, and through worship services and the use of the sacraments.[119] Pastoral counselors believed that they could help psychologists heal those suffering from psychosomatic illnesses. Odenwald and VanderVeldt said that psychosomatic illnesses were proof of the wholeness of man as stated in Catholic theology.[120]

Jewish theologians accepted the concept of psychosomatic illness easily because it logically followed from their idea that man was a holistic union of body and soul.

Liebman said in 1946 that psychosomatic medicine had shown that man destroyed himself. It was necessary for man to accept and love himself with his imperfections before he could accept and love others. Once man loved himself he could love others in their uniqueness.[121] Henry Raphael Gold said that Jews were subject to psychosomatic disorders in greater numbers than the rest of the population because of their intermittent persecution throughout history and the strains of accustoming themselves to many new cultures.[122]

Religious Education and Psychological Testing

The influence of Freudian psychology on Protestant religious education in the United States was in the reorienting of religious school teaching to emphasize the message of love of self, man, and God. Authoritarian atttitudes and pressures to behave based upon fear were eliminated from the Sunday School curriculum. The child was acknowledged as being different from an adult and warranting different treatment.[123]

A. J. Meyers in 1928 asserted that while fear was formerly an effective tool, teachers of religion now regarded it as providing a negative and repressive experience. Instead, religious teachers stressed love of the good, complemented by an understanding of what constituted bad conduct and its moral danger.[124]   V. E. Marriott commented in 1929 that progressive education was good because it enabled a child to move around spontaneously helping others, and that this method was essentially moral. He thought that other methods such as catechism were no longer needed.[125]

In 1930, B. S. Winchester proposed that the church should provide an outlet for the stress and anxiety which our rapidly changing society was producing by providing a forum for the discussion of problems.[126] J. A. Charters denied that Christianity was responsible for the degrading attitude held by some towards sex.   Religious education should encourage a wholesome respect towards sex, and this positive attitude should be upheld behaviorally by parents and pastors.[127]

Religious educators became more child-centered and showed increasing familiarity with psychology.   They tried to make religious education relevant to the problems and concerns of children, instead of emphasizing religious dogma.   In terms reminiscent of the Social Gospellers, S. C. Fahs said that religious education should not just teach about God but should be oriented towards dealing with the problems faced by children of religious school age.[128]   J. M. Andrus opined in 1929 that children were "egocentric" and adults had to see things from their viewpoint in order to be successful religious education teachers.[129]   In a 1947 restatement, C. G. McCormick declared that religious education should focus on working out solutions to children's problems as part of a general philosophical emphasis on the uniqueness and self-awareness of the individual.   Other aspects of McCormick's man-centered philosophy included teaching the children to recognize, communicate, and accept their emotions.   The child should be taught to think about God as he was revealed in the child's expressions.[130]

William B. Terhune also advocated a holistic humanistic philosphy as the basis of religious education. He advised against teaching children rigid concepts or to repress rather than direct their emotions.   He opposed an authoritarian approach in the classroom, because he thought that religion should be supportive. He wanted to discover people's needs and help them find a philosophy of life useful in solving current problems.[131]

In 1949, Ernest M. Ligon suggested that all types of psychology, including neo-Freudian psychology, should be surveyed to determine whether they could make any contribution to religious education.[132]   Ten years later, Roy A. Burkhart developed this into the idea that the church should develop an educational program about marriage and family life which would teach parents about the psychosexual states of Freudian psychology through which children passed. Parents should be taught that children passed through an oral period in the first one and one-half years, during which the child began to acquire a sense of selfhood. He then moved through an anal phase from age one and one-half to three years, in which children began to interact with others. In the genital period which lasted from age three to age five, the child began to realize the differences in his two parents.[133]

Support came from diffuse sources. Walter Houston Clark said that the roots of religious education were in love; that is, in the need to receive and give love. Love and cooperation were necessary for the success of a religious education program.[134] In the same year Stuart M. Finch and Edwin H. Kroor declared that religious education must strengthen the ego and not the superego. It was the concept of the self, not the conscience, that had to be strengthened in religious education.[135]

Catholic education was influenced by Freudian and neo-Freudian psychology chiefly in the areas of testing and guidance. Psychological tests were administered in parochial schools, and guidance services were made available to students whenever funding permitted. There was an increased emphasis upon the importance of a positive self-image among the students and of praise as a motivating tool in education.

Catholics favored the concept of guidance, which they saw as being educative rather than analytic. Guidance counselors dealt with the conscious mind and could easily direct discussions away from topics which had moral dangers for Catholics. The profession of guidance counselor began in the school, but Catholics extended the guidance function beyond the parochial school to people in religious life and especially leaders of religious life.[136]

As early as 1939 Catholics showed interest in the guidance movement. They participated in a Work Progress Administration Program to establish guidance services in parochial schools.[137] However, lack of funds prevented the rapid extension of guidance programs.[138] Catholic schools experimented with individual and group counseling techniques, often utilizing existing faculty and staff in the new counseling roles.[139] By 1965, they considered themselves to be fifteen years beyond the public school system in providing guidance services.[140]

Psychology courses were offered in Catholic high schools, colleges and nursing schools.[141] Catholics were interested in training Catholics as clinical psychologists and psychiatrists so that they could refer Catholics who needed psychotherapy to practicing psychotherapists.

Psychological concepts did not effect a major change in Jewish religious school education, which tried to give Jewish children a sense of belonging to a group and at the same time ease their adjustment to a Christian environment. They tried to teach religion through concrete experiences, not through discussions of abstract principles. They used religious ritual to inculcate Jewish values.[142]

Boris Levinson discussed the special problems of Yeshiva students. He said that the children scored very high on intelligence tests because of their superior verbal ability. He noted the emphasis Jewish culture placed on learning and said that the pressure on the children for intellectual achievement imposed a special burden on those who were less able.[143]

Testing programs were begun by religious workers much earlier than programs in pastoral counseling. Testing had many advantages over depth analysis in the eyes of religionists. Tests were scientific. They measured attitudes or abilities according to pre-established rating scales and norms which provided independent verification of the testors' findings. It was hoped that by compiling the scores and profiles of many tests it would be possible to understand the functioning of the entire human being without having to utilize theories based upon the perceptions of the therapist.

Many tests could be administered to groups of people at the same time. They were very useful for screening for traits which were desirable or undersirable. Group tests of attitudes and interests could also be used to evaluate the effectiveness of specific religious education programs which were designed to change attitudes. Some tests, such as the Rorschach Test, delved more deeply into the psyche than others, but all tested the conscious mind and were less threatening to religious people, who feared delving into the unconscious.

Although religious groups began testing programs in the 1930s, once again it was World War II which caused the boom in testing. The armed forces trained clinical psychologists to administer psychological tests, and after World War II, there were many clinical psychologists. Thus, the United States government helped to bridge the gap that had developed between experimental and behaviorist psychologists and clinical psychologists. The tests which were employed were designed by the former and used for purposes of screening and evaluating programs in which the latter were involved.

Diagnostic tests were used extensively, often as a prelude to analytic therapy, in the post–World War II period.[144] Although none of the tests could be considered as purely Freudian or neo-Freudian, some of the projective instruments like the Thematic Apperception Test or the Rorschach did require considerable interpretation by the testor and were designed to give a fairly accurate picture of the emotional life of the testee.

In the decade of the 1920s Protestants began testing to determine the attitudes of people toward religion. The purpose of the testing was to improve the effectiveness of the religious education program by determining the kinds of experiences which most often led to development of high moral character and religiosity.[145] Little testing was done in the 1930s, probably because of the difficulty in securing funds to cover the cost of research during the great depression. The subject matter of the few studies that were completed closely resembled that of the 1920s.[146] In the 1940s attempts were made to discover those factors and attitudes which led to increased religiosity in children and in adults.[147]

In the 1950s, Protestants continued to test for the origin and nature of religious attitudes.[148] Ministers began administering batteries of psychological tests as part of their pastoral counseling.[149] In addition, Protestant clerics began testing seminarians themselves to screen candidates for the ministry.[150] The use of testing expanded greatly in the 1960s. Protestant ministers screened missionary and seminary candidates for emotional stability.[151] They continued to learn about testing and to use psychological tests in pastoral counseling.[152] They tested to determine the effectiveness of courses in changing the attitudes of seminarians.[153]

Protestants continued to test to determine the cause and nature of religious belief and identification and the relationship of religious belief to other attitudes.[154] They also began to examine the attitudes and characteristics of people who had conversion experiences.[155]

Although Catholics were extremely wary of analytic clinical psychology, they were quite willing to use psychological tests to evaluate programs and look for attitudes which would lead to increased spirituality. They were interested in screening all candidates for religious life, although they cautioned that the tests provided only one kind of information that went into the judgment about the suitability of a candidate for religious life.

Although Catholics began testing attitudes somewhat later than the Protestants, they commenced testing people in religious life earlier, which probably indicated the awareness of mental health problems among those in religious life. By the 1940s Catholics were testing to determine which traits were undesirable in nuns, priets, and seminarians.[156] In the 1950s, Catholics continued screening candidates for religious life, often combining the testing with psychiatric interviews.[157]

Catholic parochial school systems developed guidance facilities and used some psychological tests like the Minnesota Multiphasic Personality Inventory Test.[158] They also made referrals of mentally ill students to psychiatrists and psychologists.[159] In the 1960s the amount of testing done in Catholic religious and educational institutions rose sharply.

Catholic educators and guidance counselors placed increased emphasis on good interpersonal relations and self-esteem.[160] Catholics expanded the testing and guidance program for people in religious life[161] and in parochial schools.[162]

The respect in which psychological tests as evaluation techniques were held was made evident when Alan K. Greenwald in 1964 insisted that reports of psychological tests should be discussed with seminarians before they were presented to their superiors.[163] Catholics continued to test for religious attitudes in order to find methods of increasing religiosity.[164]

Although some of the surveys of Jewish attitudes were sponsored by the organization of Reform congregations in the United States (the Union of American Hebrew Congregations), most of the testing was done by Jewish cultural or welfare organizations. Testing like other social services grew up outside of the synagogue.

Jewish parochial schools were few in numbers in comparison with the Catholic system, but both Orthodox Yeshivas and Conservative Jewish Day schools used psychological testing and guidance services to the extent that they were available through government programs. Few if any had the resources to offer guidance or psychological testing programs independently.

Testing of Jewish students was designed to pinpoint those characteristics, attitudes, and interests which could be considered as particularly Jewish, leading to the identification of Jews with their cultural and religious heritage.[165] Jews also sought to identify those aspects of Jewish and Christian culture[166] which seemed to favor the development of anti-semitic attitudes. The earliest studies were done in the 1930s and the same areas were investigated through to the 1960s.

Influence of Psychology on Religion, 1965–1978

In the years following 1965, the pattern already set was not altered in any significant way, so far as religion and its response are concerned. The reconciliation of Freudian and neo-Freudian psychology and religion continued. The testing of ministerial candidates also continued, as did comparisons of religious and non-religious people.[1] Robert L. Williams and Cole Spurgion investigated Freud's theory that religion was the result of insecurity, by measuring anxiety over death according to a test rating scale of their own design.[2] Other psychologists tried to develop a test to measure religious neuroticism and to measure the degree of regression that occurred in intense conversion experience.[3]

Theologians analyzed religious figures in psychological terms.[4] They expressed a more naturalistic view of sex. Andrew R. Eickhoff discussed St. Paul's sexual attitudes. He argued that St. Paul lived in a male-dominated society where all women were submissive. St. Paul considered that mode of social organization as God-ordained. He viewed women as sexual temptresses whose own sex drives were diffuse. He said that abstinence, sublimation, and repression of the sex drive was preferable to the problems of marriage. Eickhoff disagreed. He pronounced St. Paul immoderate and ignorant of the expression of the sex drive in sadism and in repression.[5] Protestant ministers continued to give pastoral counseling which increasingly resembled psychotherapy.[6]

Pastoral theology was a pragmatic mixture of Freudian and neo-Freudian psychology and Christianity. The ministry developed techniques for dealing with specific problems such as patients suffering from cancer.[7] J. Stanley Glen criticized neo-Freudian psychology from the perspective of the 1960s. He concluded that Fromm reflected the concerns of the 1930s about the role of deterministic totalitarian ideologies; Fromm found the Christian gospel wanting for vesting power in God rather than in man. Since he distrusted any authoritarian philosophy, Fromm misunderstood the paradox of divine grace which was revolutionary and reactionary at the same time.[8]

Clergymen went on working in community mental health centers.[9] They still tried to combine psychoanalytic techniques with parochial functions to develop new educational programs.[10] Protestants continued to be very interested in the phenomena of religious conversion. Joel Allison said that recent studies showed that most conversions were not regressive and were not similar to schizophrenia.[11] Most converts enjoyed good interpersonal relations.

Catholics were still cautiously examining psychology in order to determine which elements were compatible with the teachings of the church. Andre Godin warned of the special difficulties which transference neuroses posed for priests who might be tempted to seek out the type of counselee with whom they could easily establish a transference relationship.[12] Carlo Weber, a psychotherapist who treated nuns and priests, said that prayers and rituals formed such an important part of Catholicism that they were felt to be dehumanizing by some people in religious life. Weber noted that the three vows of poverty, chastity, and obedience which were taken by a person in religious life could be used to escape from human contact and avoid responsibility for one's actions. Religious life could bring depersonalization and operant conditioning, with a resultant loss of identity. Weber felt that the "caste system" and the judgmental attitude in the church were damaging to the individual.[13]

Sharon MacIsaacs showed the similarities between Freud's theory of the sexual drive as the motivating force of the unconscious and the Catholic doctrine of original sin. She asserted that, according to the doctrine of original sin, man was divided within himself and was "formed by his environment at a level anterior to his choice."[14] Sin or sexual lust caused self-alienation in man. MacIsaacs said that the sexual instincts could not be entirely controlled because they existed both on an unconscious and on a conscious level. The ego was not the controlling force in the personality; it only seemed to come under control through "incomplete and untrustworthy perceptions."[15] Therefore, original sin should be thought of as a general alienation of self rather than a narrow sexual lust.

MacIsaacs departed from Thomistic psychology when she said that neither the ego nor the conscious mind was master of the human personality. She also attempted to equate sin with self-alienation. The concept of sin as being untrue to one's self, one's spirituality or one's goals, had been suggested earlier by both Protestant and Jewish theologians.

Vincent V. Heir reported on mental health programs for seminarians. He said that the program involved preventive work in mental health, referrals to other agencies, the development of techniques for training laymen as mental health workers and helping people achieve well-adjusted personalities.[16] Le Roy A. Warwick discussed the problems of Catholic clergymen functioning as marriage counselors, the most common problem for which people consulted clergymen.[17]

The role of the minister was continuing to change during the 1970s. Catholic priests were studying parish psychology in order to become more effective pastoral counselors. Catholics emphasized the importance of loving and of sharing and tried to be less directive.

Jewish theologians were increasingly aware of the contributions that the insights of psychology could make to their understanding of the human psyche. More and more rabbis took courses in psychology and in techniques of counseling. They understood Freud's philosophy as an outgrowth of the era in which he lived and something which could be readily separated from his dynamic psychology. Jack Bemporad felt that Freud ignored the emotional sustenance offered by religion. Repentance, which had to be a "primary process," had the ability to change the past and the future because no meanings were absolutely sure until the end of history.[18] Bemporad said that God existed independently of man. He agreed with Fromm's differentiation of humanistic from authoritarian religion in *Psychoanalysis and Religion*.[19]

In all branches of religion the adaptation of psychological concepts to religious uses continued as contemporary American culture became increasingly influenced by the "triumph of the therapeutic."[20]

In the Progressive Era, the beginning period for this study, there was no awareness of Freudian or of post-Freudian theory among theologians. Sixty-five years later, the influence of Freudian and post-Freudian theory and practice upon religion in America was substantial, especially in the areas of ministerial education and pastoral practice.

During the first decades of the twentieth century there was a gradual increase in awareness of Freudian theory and psychoanalytic practice, derived from popular journals of opinion, movies, and the theater; also, translations of Freud's writings were becoming available in the United States. Concurrently there was an increase in the use of Freudian analytic and therapeutic techniques on these shores.

However, religious leaders did not express much interest in Freud's ideas, if one is to judge by the religious journals of the time. An exception was a degree of positive response by pastors working in institutions. Early comment on Freud appearing in religious journals tended to have a negative and even derisive tone, and to indicate greater familiarity with his later works, which were more concerned with social psychology and with anthropology than with psychoanalytic theory or technique.

With the exception of the clinical training programs, which were most often serving those who had chosen to assume an institutional ministry, there was little interest in psychology in American religious circles before World War II.

There were many reasons why this was the case. Freudian theory was generally not very attractive to clergymen. Freud had dethroned rational man while exalting the role of the libido, and the reproductive instincts in particular, in human behavior. He described the Oedipus complex in great detail while leaving the measure of control an individual could exercise over his behavior, and hence, the degree to which he could be held responsible for it, in great doubt. In addition, most of Freud's social and anthropological speculations were in conflict with traditional religious views about the origin and nature of society. Furthermore, Freud treated religious figures like Moses and Jesus Christ in an irreverent manner. As yet, Freud's aesthetic, materialistic outlook was enough to convince most theologians that there was nothing in his psychology which merited their attention.

The post-Freudians, like Sullivan, Fromm, and Horney, received a warmer welcome from theologians. These later theorists came after the initial shock caused by Freudian theory had been somewhat absorbed. They were writing during a period of greater social crisis when the need for and advances in the art of mental healing was more widely apparent, and they concentrated on ego psychology and the importance of interpersonal relations to mental health, a concept familiar to pastors. Although post-Freudians also tended to be atheists, on the whole they spoke more positively about organized religion. However, World War II caused both psychologists and religionists to reconsider their positions. Ministers felt that they were not successfully able to deal with current social problems by traditional methods, while psychologists were so distressed by wartime atrocities and domestic social problems that they re-examined the socializing role played by organized religion. Although their statements about the existence of God still gave little comfort to religionists, they did find merit in religious fellowship and practices. Thus, a truce was struck between two warring camps. Although critical articles continued to appear in Catholic and Protestant lay magazines like *Christian Century*, those religionists who did not support the new pastoral psychology, seem to have directed their attention elsewhere. Similarly, the science versus religion argument to which psychology was sometimes joined, seemed to abate, although there continued to be skirmishes. In a technocratic atomic age, few Americans denigrated science, and social scientists seemed more interested in investigating religion than in lambasting it. In addition, once one side realized that the other was no longer firing off polemics, it too tended to desist and let a productive dialogue develop.

The decade of the 1950s was crucial for the acceptance of Freudian and neo-Freudian psychology by organized religion, although some agitation for a synthesis of psychology and religion to be used in pastoral counseling had begun before among institutional chaplains before World War II. Ministers who had received clinical training while serving as armed forces chaplains, and who had found the traditional religious practices inadequate for dealing with the mental problems which developed during wartime, returned home and used the same clinical insights and techniques in dealing with problems at home.

During the 1950s, pastoral psychology was synthesized at home from the intellectual contributions of European-born native analysts whose insights were applied to traditional Judeo-Christian thought by theologians and psychologists.

It held greater appeal for those theologians and pastors whose outlook could be termed as rational, scientific, and group-oriented as opposed to those who tended to be more romantic, pietistic, and individualistic. Although Freud himself was interested in philosophy and engaged in anthropological speculation, his method and training were scientific.

After World War II, existentialist psychologists and theologians like Paul Tillich and O. Hobart Mowrer offered intellectual syntheses of existentialist psychology and theology which appeared in the journals of pastoral psychology. Although the syntheses were interesting they offered little in the way of practical help for the counseling pastor, and hence, were of little interest to him. Ministers read articles about pastoral psychology as they searched for solutions to everyday pastoral problems. They were not very interested in theoretical syntheses.

The *Journal of Pastoral Care* and *Pastoral Psychology* were founded within five years of the end of World War II, and served as the chief organs for dissemination of Freudian and post-Freudian pastoral psychology. The most frequent contributors to these journals were the new professors of pastoral care at Protestant theological seminaries. Parish ministers with a special interest in the implications of psychology for pastoral practice were the next most common group of contributors, with about ten percent of the articles published being written by leading post-Freudian theorists. The readers of the journals were hard-working ministers with pastoral problems to which denominational journals paid little attention. Beyond a doubt, these two journals greatly increased pastoral awareness of and receptivity to Freudian insights.

Postwar clerics, finding themselves less successful as pastors than before, were willing to learn new techniques by which they could improve their effectiveness as pastoral counselors and as ministers of God. They viewed clinical techniques as another weapon in their arsenal, which they could use to bring man closer to God. Theologians received help from the leading neo-Freudians as well as from mental health workers of all kinds in reformulating theological concepts and adapting pastoral practices for greater validity.

Both ministers and psychologists stated emphatically that psychology did not offer a substitute for religion and that the practice of religion did not guarantee mental health. Both psychology and religion could be misused, and thereby seem to usurp the domain of the other, but this should not happen. Each should recognize and respect the contribution of the other. The religionists accepted the neo-Freudian description of man's dynamic structure, and psychologists tried to avoid making definitive statements about the existence of God. Ministers pointed out, and at times exaggerated, those aspects of traditional psychology which seemed to be especially psychologically valid, and psychologists were generous in their praise of those aspects of religion which they considered to be psychologically supportive.

The three major religious groups were affected differently by Freudian and neo-Freudian psychology. The greatest change occurred in liberal Protestantism, where theological concepts, the education of ministers, and the entire concept of pastoral care changed.

Liberal Protestantism led in the acceptance of Freudian and post-Freudian theory because they were the only liberal group whose member assumed an extensive pastoral role, and hence had a greater need for better ways to treat mental health problems.

Reform Judaism was similarly affected but to a lesser degree, because Jewish social service institutions developed outside of the synagogue, and the rabbi normally did little pastoral counseling. Indeed, the Jewish response to psychology occurred in the social service, not the religious journals. Therefore, although his psychological orientation was similar to that of the liberal Protestant minister, the total impact of pastoral psychology on his rabbinical activities was not great. Orthodox Jewish religious practices remained almost totally unaffected by psychology, although Orthodox Jews were treated by psychotherapists.

Catholic clergymen were constrained from widespread acceptance by their conservatism, their acceptance of Thomistic psychology, and their reluctance to re-examine their attitudes towards sex in the light of modern psychology. They did, however, emphasize the importance of acting out of love, not fear. Fundamentalist and pentecostal sects seemed to ignore this development in pastoral psychology.

Catholic social service agencies, like Catholic Charities, existed outside of the Church. Cries for the acceptance of psychology arose first from Catholic institutional chaplains and next from those working in Catholic social service agencies, but they were not heeded by the Catholic clergy in general.

The reasons for the reluctance of Catholic clergy, in particular, and some Protestant clergymen to delay or deny acceptance of psychology included Freud's atheism and materialistic philosophy and the anti-religious attitudes he expressed in works such as *The Future of an Illusion* and *Totem and Taboo*. Catholic clergymen believed that the teachings of the Church could not be modified according to any new set of ideas. It was the new material which had to conform to the teachings of the Church. In addition, both Catholic and conservative Protestant clergymen were concerned that the acceptance of psychotherapeutic, non-judgmental attitudes would undermine the moral basis of society. All of these factors resulted in very limited acceptance of psychology by Catholics and by conservative Protestants.

All religionists were happiest when they discovered that traditional religious practices were psychologically valid. The concurrence of Protestant and Jewish emphasis on the importance of fellowship and love with neo-Freudian emphasis on self-love and self-acceptance and the importance of good object relations in the development of an individual is a case in point. Similarly, traditional Jewish mourning practices seemed, to reform theologians, to be psychologically valid. In other cases, theologians were willing to give questionable emphasis to citations from ancient sources to prove traditional thought was valid in terms of modern psychology. Jewish theologians seemed especially prone to this type of over-emphasis, although theologians from all three groups were guilty to some extent. Psychology also had offered new interpretations of man's behavior which made some traditional forms of religious behavior seem less desirable.

Protestant denominations like Presbyterians, Methodists, Episco-palians, and Southern Baptists, along with more intellectual Catholics and secularly educated Jews were the most interested in pastoral psychology. There was no evidence in the literature of interest by groups which could be considered to be basically fundamentalist or pentecostal in outlook. The movement seemed have to affected those with a more modern and perhaps urban outlook.

Pastoral counseling occasionally took slightly different forms. Where ministers became involved in the community mental health movement, pastoral psychologists were likely to work in interdenomi-national, clerical or lay community counseling centers, where such existed, in addition to bringing a psychological orientation to their parish counseling and fellowship activities. Where no community counseling centers existed, the minister might have an informal working relationship with other mental health professionals to whom he might make referrals. Naturally, since the clinical training movement had always been an interdenominational movement in which laymen exerted great influence, the ability to feel comfortable in an ecumenical and mixed lay and clerical environment was almost a necessity.

In the 1950s there was thorough re-examination of the problems of guilt and anxiety, with significant use of psychological understandings about the nature of guilt and anxiety and the problem of assessing man's ultimate responsibility for his actions. Recognition of the problems of neurotic guilt and of scrupulosity, and of the total lack of guilt as indicative of mental illness, represented areas where theology deliberately strove to incorporate psychology in order to further mental health.

Theologians were interested in exploring the nature and effect of anxiety upon the individual. Theologians and psychologists often differed about the existence of anxiety and about man's relationship with God as a distinct and a healthy form of anxiety, but they were otherwise in agreement about the reality of both guilt and anxiety and the usefulness of these emotions in helping man control his behavior. With the exception of what theologians called anxiety about "the holy dread," traditional theology and psychological theory blended on the subject of guilt and anxiety. There was no reformulation of religious concepts of guilt and anxiety. The ministers rarely used their new therapeutic skills to try to deal with guilt and anxiety among parishioners. Salvation remained the ultimate goal of the minister, although he might borrow from the social sciences to bring people closer to the divine. That crucial last step towards salvation was still to be made in a fairly traditional manner, possibly with less emphasis on man's unworthiness.

Another important change was the stress on the necessity of self-love and self-acceptance which had to precede love of others and of God. This was accompanied by a general elevation of the worshipper from a debased sinner to a human capable of great love and joyful striving to fulfill God's commandments, who could accept God's forgiveness as the culmination of his efforts to love and to accept himself, his fellow man and God. Catholics retained the traditional formulation of love of God as primary followed by love of others at the same intensity as self-love, although they stressed the importance of love as a motivating force.

The amending of the commandment to love God, to the effect that man had to first be able to love himself and his fellow man before he could expect to be able to love God, represented one of the few real theological modifications in a religious theory as the result of the influence of Freudian and post-Freudian psychology.   Another theological change among Protestants and Conservative and Reform Jews was the acceptance of man as an essentially irrational creature instead of one who was the possessor of reason.   Catholics and Orthodox Jews retained the traditional view of man as having reason and free will, but in practice Catholics recognized that neuroses, psychoses, and other mental disorders limited the operation of free will and the degree of sin that could result from actions committed by a person with impaired reason.   Thus, although they maintained that man had free will, they acknowledged in practice that a significant segment of the population did not have the capacity to utilize their free will and reason, and their actions were greatly determined by forces which were beyond their conscious control.   In addition, theologians no longer greeted all conversion experiences with a resounding *hallelujah!*   Instead, they looked for empirical evidence in the subsequent behavior of the convert as to whether he was experiencing divine grace or mental illness.

In other cases theologians seemed to rationalize existing changes. More relaxed sexual attitudes were examples of this kind of change. Theologians of all faiths approved of sexuality within marriage. They did not approve of extramarital sexual activity, although even Catholics stressed the poor rate of success of pastors who worked to reform the practices of homosexuals or chronic masturbators.   Thus, while maintaining that those activities were mortal sins, they seemed to grant them some grudging acceptance.

Although theological reformulations were rare, pastoral practice did change, taking on a therapeutic, in place of an authoritarian, complexion. Ministers were most receptive to change in counseling techniques in order to become more effective pastors of their flocks, and in particular, to be able to deal more effectively with the acute counseling problems presented by alcoholics, the divorced, the bereaved, and the mentally ill. Besides being interested in the dynamics of personality which were involved in problems such as alcoholism, ministers tried to modify their approach to all counselees in order to be less authoritarian, more non-directive and generally more accepting.   Although they felt that ultimately a minister had to render a moral judgment when God's law was being broken, he could defer pronouncng the judgment until he felt that the counselee was sufficiently un-alienated and could accept it. Some ministers found therapeutic techniques such as group therapy ideally suited to and in effect paralleling existing church practice.

The greatest impact of psychology on religion occurred in the field of the clinical training of ministers.   Most of the leaders of the movement for the incorporation of psychotherapeutic techniques and understandings into theology and religious practice were part of the clinical training movement. Men like Anton T. Boisen, the father of clinical training who founded the first clinical training programs for ministers, and Philip Guiles, who founded the Institute For Pastoral Care and became the supervising institutional chaplain in clinical training programs, pioneered in applying therapeutic techniques and psychological insights to the counseling ministry. Later leaders like Seward Hiltner, David Roberts, Wayne Oates, and Paul Johnson were all frequent contributors to the psychologically-oriented journals of pastoral care, and were professors of pastoral psychology in Protestant seminaries. Others, like Ernest Bruder, continued to serve and to train others as hospital chaplains. Although these men were Protestant clergymen and the clinical training movement was dominated by Protestants, Jewish and Catholic groups sponsored some training programs.

The ministers who led the clinical training programs often assumed professorships in theological seminaries, from which they declared that a minister had to understand Freudian and neo-Freudian psychology in order to be able to give adequate pastoral care to parishioners. They also led the movement to make clinical training part of every minister's education, and provided part-time and full-time programs for ordained ministers and for seminarians. Thus, pastoral psychology was taught to the young and old during the same time period and represented a significant change in clerical education. Although the clinical training movement was strongest in Protestantism, similar developments occurred in Catholicism and in Reform and Conservative Judaism. Professors of pastoral psychology dispensed advice about the theory and practice of Freudian and neo-Freudian psychology as applied to pastoral problems. Their view of man changed; sickness was equated with sin and righteous living with mental health. Ministerial views of anxiety, guilt, and sexuality were also to become more sophisticated while all of theology was scrutinized as to its psychological validity. Although there was some feeling that every pastoral contact should utilize neo-Freudian techniques of counseling, there were no suggestions in the literature that everyone was to some extent sick, and in need of therapy.

The leaders in the clinical training movement were affiliated with the major theological seminaries, which would normally be less conservative than those without a major university affiliation. The movement was strongest throughout the Northeast, the mid-Atlantic states and states of the old Northwest Territory. Ministers from predominantly rural areas like the deep South, the West, and the Southwest and the Pacific coast seemed to be less involved, although the movement did spread to the urban west during the late 1960s and 1970s. The West coast was a special case; there, an abundance of psychological self-help and positive thinking groups which made therapy easily available to most people probably allowed organized religion to pay less attention to psychology. People interested in the psychological approach to their problems could easily find that kind of care elsewhere. Ministers in rural areas, where the traditional familial and fraternal organizations remained stronger, faced fewer social problems such as divorce and juvenile delinquency. Thus, there was less need for new remedies in rural society.

Another influence of psychology upon religious education was the use of psychological tests. They were most often used to test for the existence of and possible changes in religious attitudes. Projective psychological tests were also used to screen candidates for the ministry, seminary candidates, and those wishing to enter religious life.

Religion as a supportive socializing force in American life has probably benefited from the acceptance of psychological theory. The use of therapeutic techniques probably made ministers more effective as counselors while it did not noticeably detract from their priestly function. The clinical training which ministers received might aid them in the recognition of the onset of serious mental problems in parishioners in localities where few if any other mental health services were available. Whether psychotherapy was in truth an aid to salvation cannot really be said.

Since one of the uses of religion to society was to enforce moral standards, the adoption of a therapeutic non-judgmental morality would probably not strengthen the bonds which united any society and would rob religion of part of its unique contribution, the establishment of a code of ethics.

The political temper of the times was another aid to the proponents of pastoral psychology. The battle for the acceptance of Freudian and neo-Freudian psychology was fought and won in the 1950s when the rival materialist ideology, Marxism, was in great disrepute in the United States. Proponents of Marxism believed that man's behavior could be understood in terms of his seeking to satisfy his economic needs. Freudian psychologists considered the biological libidinal drives which were housed in the Freudian id as the determinants of man's behavior. Individualists, irrational Freudian man stood in sharp contrast to collectivist, economically determined Marxian man, and the neo-Freudian de-emphasis of the sexual drive and increased emphasis on interpersonal relations did not lessen the contrast between psychology and socialism. In addition, in the anti-communist American political climate of the

1950s, all collectivist ideologies seemed unattractive. The structure of the family and of the society in general seemed to be disintegrating at a previously unheard-of rate, but the economy remained relatively sound. Therefore, other social scientists voiced little opposition to theories of psychological motivation. Neither did they offer alternative solutions to contemporary problems. Americans seemed to need therapy, not economic reorganization, and many ministers of all faiths tried to respond with a religion which was psychologically valid. To a great extent, liberal American religion could not resist the pressures which were developing for a culture which would be uniformly therapeutic.

Notes

Chapter One

1. Nathan G. Hale, *Freud and the Americans: The Beginnings of Psychoanalysis in the United States, 1876-1917* (New York: Oxford University Press, 1971), pp. 4-5.

2. Edwin G. Boring, *History of Experimental Psychology*, 2nd ed. (New York: Appleton-Century-Crofts, 1950), p. 506.

3. William James, *Varieties of Religious Experience* (New York: Random House, Inc., 1929).

4. Ibid., p. 202.

5. Ibid., p. 197.

6. P. Franklin, "Measurement of the Comprehensive Difficulty of the Precepts and Parables of Jesus," *University of Iowa Studies: Studies in Character* 2, no. 1, (1967) p. 63.

7. E. D. Starbuck, "An Empirical Study of Mysticism," *Proceedings of the Sixth International Congress on Philosophy* (New York: Longmans Green, 1926), pp. 87-94.

8. R. H. Thouless, "Scientific Method in the Study of Psychology of Religion," *Character and Personality* 7 (1938): 103-8.

9. Hale, p. 52.

Chapter Two

1. Ernest Jones, *The Life and Work of Sigmund Freud*, ed. L. Trilling and S. Marcus (New York: Basic Books, 1961).

2. In addition to the basic works of Sigmund Freud, which will be mentioned throughout the chapter, the following secondary sources have been used: *The Basic Writings of Sigmund Freud*, ed. A. A. Brill (New York: Modern Library, Random House, 1938); Reuben Fine, *Freud: A Critical Re-Evaluation of His Theories* (New York: David McKay Co., 1962); Calvin S. Hall and Gardiner Lindzey, *Theories of Personality* (New York: John Wiley & Sons, 1957); Silvano Arieti, ed., *American Handbook of Psychiatry*, vol. 1 (New York: Basic Books, 1974), ch. 37.

3. Charles Darwin, *On the Origin of Species.* (Chicago: Encyclopedia Britannica Press, 1955).

Chapter Three

1. Arieti, pp. 789-808; James A.C. Brown, *Freud and the Post Freudians* (London: Penguin Books, Ltd., 1974), pp. 41-42.

2. Arieti, pp. 809-18; Brown, pp. 42-49; Paul Roazan, *Freud and His Followers* (New York: Alfred A. Knopf, 1975), pp. 224-76.

3. Arieti, pp. 914-19; Brown, pp. 392-405; Roazan, pp. 53-54.

4. Arieti, pp. 819-27; Brown, pp. 67-78; Roazan, pp. 457-58.

5. Arieti, pp. 442-57; Brown, pp. 77-78; Roazan, pp. 68-71.

6. Arieti, pp. 828-42; Brown, pp. 82-86.

7. Arieti, pp. 843-53; Brown, pp. 165-73.

8. Arieti, p. 904; Brown, pp. 100-3; Roazan, pp. 503-4.

9. Arieti, pp. 862-76; Brown, pp. 129-48.

10. Arieti, pp. 843-60; Brown, pp. 149-63.

Chapter Four

1. Jacob A. Arlow, "A Psychoanalytic Study of a Religious Initiation Rite: Bar Mitzvah," in Ruth S. Eissler, et al. *The Psychoanalytic Study of the Child* 4 (1927): 353-74.

2. Róheim, G., "Animism and Religion," *Psychoanalytic Quarterly* 1 (1932): 59-112.

3. Margaret Mead, *Coming of Age in Samoa* (New York: Mentor, 1963); Bronislaw Malinowski, *Argonauts of the Western Pacific* (New York: Dutton, 1961).

4. J. B. Holt, "Holiness Religion: Cultural Shock and Social Reorganization," *American Sociological Review* 5 (1940): 740-47.

5. E. M. Rosenzweig, "Minister and Congregation – A Study in Ambivalence," *Psychoanalytic Review* 28 (1941): 218-27.

6. J. M. Mecklin, *The Passing of the Saint: A Study of a Cultural Type* (Chicago: University Press, 1941).

7. Hans Sachs, "At the Gates of Heaven," *American Imago* 4 (1947): 15-32.

8. Jacob Taubes, "Religion and the Future of Psychoanalysis," *Psychoanalysis* 4 (1957): 136-42.

9. Herbert Moller, "Affective Mysticism in Western Civilization," *Psychoanalytic Review* 52 (1965): 115-30.

10. Lewis A. Rhodes, "Authoritarianism and Fundamentalism of Rural and Urban High School Students," *Journal of Educational Sociology* 34 (1960): 97-105.

11. Perry Londin, et al., "Religion, Guilt and Ethical Standards," *Journal of Social Psychology* 63 (December 1964): 145-59.

12. Charles T. O'Reilly and Edward J. O'Reilly, "Religious Beliefs of Catholic College Students and Their Attitudes Towards Minoritism," *Journal of Abnormal Social Psychology* 4 (1954): 378-80.

13. Mortimer Ostow, "The Nature of Religious Controls," *American Psychologist* 13 (1958): 71-74.

Chapter Five

1. P. McW. Grant, "The Moral and Religious Life of the Individual in the Light of the New Psychology." *Mental Hygiene* 12 (1928): 449-91.

2. W. A. R. Leys, "Soul Saving in the Light of Modern Psychology," *Religious Education* 25 (1930): 344-49.

3. Anton T. Boisen, *The Exploration of the Inner World: A Study of Mental Disorder and Religious Experience* (Chicago: Willett Clark, 1936).

4. E. B. Backus, "Religion and Mental Health," *Mental Hygiene Review* 1 (1940):14-18.

5. Seward Hiltner, "The Contributions of Religion to Mental Health," *Mental Hygiene* 24 (1940): 366-77.

6. K. R. Stolz, *The Church and Psychotherapy* (New York: Abingdon Cokesbury Press, 1943).

7. Carney P. Landis, "Psychotherapy and Religion," *Review of Religion* 10 (1946): 413-24.

8. Editorial, *Journal of Pastoral Care* 1 (Winter 1947): 33.

9. David E. Roberts, "Theological and Psychiatric Interpretations of Human Nature," *Journal of Pastoral Care* 1 (Winter 1947): 11-18.

10. Carney P. Landis, "Psychotherapy and Religion," *Journal of Pastoral Care* 1 (Spring-Summer 1947): 19-27.

11. Rollin J. Fairbanks, "Cooperation Between Clergy and Psychiatrists," *Journal of Pastoral Care* 1 (Spring-Summer 1947): 5-11.

12. Albert Outler, "Christian Context for Counseling," *Journal of Pastoral Care* 2 (Spring 1948): 1-12.

13. The *Journal of Clinical Pastoral Work* merged with the *Journal of Pastoral Care* as of the Spring-Summer issue of 1950. The Council for Clinical Training, an

association dedicated to the clinical training of ministers, was responsible for its publicaticn.

14.   David E. Roberts, *Psychotherapy and a Christian View of Man* (New York: Chas. Scribner's & Sons, 1950).

15.   Sigmund Freud, *The Psychopathology of Everyday Life.*

16.   Seward Hiltner, "Religion and Psychoanalysis," *Journal of Pastoral Care* 3 (Spring-Summer 1950): 32-42.

17.   Lawrence S. Kubic, "Psychoanalysis and Healing by Faith," *Pastoral Psychology* 1 (March 1950): 13-18.

18.   Lloyd E. Foster, "Religion and Psychiatry," *Pastoral Psychology* 1 (February 1950): 7-13.

19.   "What can the minister reasonably expect from a psychiatrist or psychologist in terms of the latter's dealing with moral principles in the life of his patient?" *Pastoral Psychology* 1 (March 1950): 55-56.

20.   Wayne E. Oates, Review of *Christianity and Fear: A Study in History* and *The Psychology and Hygiene of Religion*, by Oskar Pfister, trans. W. H. Johnston, *Pastoral Psychology* 1 (February 1950): 61-63.

21.   Paul Luschermer, "Responsibility and Its Relation to Personality Problems," *Pastoral Psychology* 1 (May 1950): 16-22.

22.   Karl Menninger, "Religion and Psychiatry," *Pastoral Psychology* 2 (September 1951): 10-18.

23.   Seward Hiltner, "Pastoral Psychology and Pastoral Counseling," *Pastoral Psychology* 3 (November 1952): 21-28.

24.   T. J. Bingham, "Moral Responsibility of the Parishioner or Patient," *Journal of Pastoral Care* 6 no. 1 (1952): 46-55.

25.   Rollo May, "Religion: Source of Strength or Weakness," *Pastoral Psychology* 4 (February 1953): 68-73.

26.   Albert Outler, *Psychotherapy and the Christian Message* (New York: Harper & Brothers, 1954).

27.   Ibid., p. 142.

28.   Ibid., p. 144.

29.   Ibid., p. 201.

30.   Ibid., p. 82.

31. W. Bonaro Overstreet, "The Unloving Personality and Religion of Love," *Pastoral Psychology* 4 (May 1953): 14-20.

32. Roy A. Burkhart, "Is the Church Authoritarian?" *Pastoral Psychology* 5 (April 1954): 25-28.

33. Carl Binger, "Moral Implications of Psychoanalysis," *Pastoral Psychology* 6 (December 1955): 19-26.

34. A. Graham, "Psychological Problems of Maturity," *Pastoral Psychology* 5 (April 1954): 47-54.

35. Wayne E. Oates, "The Helping and Hindering Power of Religion," *Pastoral Psychology* 6 (May 1955): 41-49.

36. Carroll A. Wise, *Psychiatry and the Bible* (New York: Harper & Brothers, 1956).

37. Seward Hiltner, "Freud, Psychoanalysis and Religion," *Pastoral Psychology* 7 (November 1956): 9-21.

38. For a more complete discussion of neo-Freudian theories see Chapter III.

39. Carrol Murphy, "The Ministry of Counseling," *Pastoral Psychology* 8 (December 1957): 15-32.

40. Revel L. Howe, "The Crucial and Correlative Role of Pastoral Theology," *Pastoral Psychology* 11 (February 1960): 37-44.

41. Leon D. Salzman, "Morality of Psychoanalysis," *Pastoral Psychology* 11 (March 1960): 24-29.

42. James A. Knight, "Calvinism and Psychoanalysis: A Comparative Study," *Pastoral Psychology* 13 (December 1963): 10-17.

     Another article which compared Freud and Calvin was Lawrence Frank, Review of *Life Against Death* by Norman O. Brown, *Pastoral Psychology* 10 (December 1959): 74.

43. Many authors were concerned with the themes of fellowship and growth. The following is only a representative sampling: Donald J. Butler, "Theology and Psychology: Some Points of Convergence," *Encounter*, 1958, pp. 31-46; Anton Boisen, "The Distinctive Task of the Minister," *Pastoral Psychology* 3 (April 1952): 13-15; Charles F. Golden, "Religion and Current Trends in Psychology," *Religious Education* 45 (1950): 331-35; Ernest Bruder, "Some Reflections on Psychiatry and Religion," *Journal of Pastoral Care* 5 (Summer 1951): 30-36; Edith Weigert, "Love and Fear; A Psychological Interpretation," *Journal of Pastoral Care* 5 (Summer 1951): 12-22.

44. Albert C. Outler, *Psychotherapy and the Christian Message*; Wayne E. Oates, *Religious Dimensions of Personality* (New York: Associated Press, 1957).

45. Seward Hiltner, "Religion and Psychoanalysis," *Journal of Pastoral Care* 1 (Spring-Summer 1950): 32-42; Robert A. Preston, "A Chaplain Looks at Psychiatry," *Bulletin of the Menninger Clinic* 14 (1950): 22-26; Lawrence S. Kubic, "Psychoanalysis and Healing Faith," *Pastoral Psychology* 1 (March 1950): 3-8; D. Roberts, "Co-operation Between Religion and Psychotherapy," *Pastoral Psychology* 1 (May 1950): 23-27.

46. Arieti, p. 927.

47. Paul Tillich, "Psychoanalysis, Existentialism, and Theology," *Pastoral Psychology* 9 (October 1958): 9-17.

48. Paul Tillich, "The Impact of Pastoral Psychology on Theological Thought," *Pastoral Psychology* 11 (February 1960): 17-23.

49. Carl Rogers, "Divergent Trends in Methods of Improving Adjustment," *Pastoral Psychology* 1 (September 1950): 11-18.

50. Paul E. Johnson, "Methods of Pastoral Counseling," *Journal of Pastoral Care* 1, no. 1 (1947): 27-32.

51. Rollo May, "Religion, Psychotherapy, and the Achievement of Selfhood," *Pastoral Psychology* 2 (October 1951): 29-33.

52. Rollo May, "Religion, Psychotherapy, and the Achievement of Selfhood," *Pastoral Psychology* 2 (November 1951): 15-20.

53. Rollo May, "Religion, Psychotherapy, and the Achievement of Selfhood," *Pastoral Psychology* 2 (January 1952): 26-33.

54. Rollo May, "The Healing Power of Symbols," *Pastoral Psychology* 11 (November 1960): 37-49.

55. For a fuller discussion of the development of ego psychology see Chapter III.

56. O. Hobart Mowrer, *The Crisis in Psychiatry and Religion* (Princeton: Van Nostrand, 1961).

57. Charles Stinnette, "Reflections and Transformations," in Dialogues and Comments on an Article by Alden, "Revelation and Psychotherapy," *I Continuum* 2, no. 2 (1964): 85-110.

58. Several books about existentialist pastoral psychology were reviewed in *Pastoral Psychology*. One such book was *The Doctor and the Soul* by Victor E. Frankl (New York: Alfred A. Knopf, 1956). It was reviewed by Wayne Oates in *Pastoral Psychology* 7 (June 1956): 65. Frankl called existential therapy "Logotherapy." Frankl tried to restore meaning to the lives of alienated people.

59. Seward Hiltner, Review of *Practical and Theoretical Aspects of Psychoanalysis* by Lawrence S. Kubic, *Pastoral Psychology* 1 (April 1950): 63-64.

60. Karen Horney, "The Search for Glory," *Pastoral Psychology* 1 (September 1950): 13-20.

61. Reinhold Niebuhr, "The Christian Moral Witness and some Disciplines of Modern Culture," *Pastoral Psychology* 11 (February 1960): 45-54.

62. C. W. Morris, "The Terror of Good Works," *Pastoral Psychology* 8 (July 1957): 25-32.

63. For a more complete discussion of Fromm's theories see pp. 29-31.

64. Seward Hiltner, "Pastoral Psychology and Christian Ethics," *Pastoral Psychology* 4 (April 1953): 32-33.

65. Paul Tillich, Review of *Psychoanalysis and Religion* by Erich Fromm, *Pastoral Psychology* 2 (June 1951): 62.

66. Ibid.

67. For a further discussion of Freud's philosophy see pp. 13-15.

68. Erich Fromm, "Freud and Jung," *Pastoral Psychology* 1 (July 1950): 11-15.

69. Anton T. Boisen, Letter to "Reader's Forum," *Pastoral Psychology* 2 (September 1951): 32-34.

70. Erich Fromm, "The Philosophy Basic to Freud's Psychoanalysis," *Pastoral Psychology* 13 (February 1962): 26-32.

71. Carl Jung, "Psychotherapist of the Clergy," *Pastoral Psychology* 7 (April 1956): 25-42.

72. J. Maxwell Chamberlin, "Reader's Forum," *Pastoral Psychology* (April 1956): 54.

73. Ibid., p. 55.

74. For a more complete discussion of Jung's theories see pp. 20-22.

75. Seward Hiltner, Review of *Religion and the Cure of Souls in Jung's Psychology* by Hans Schaer, trans. R. F. C. Hull, *Pastoral Psychology* (September 1950): 60-61.

76. Clara Thompson, "Towards a Psychology of Women," *Pastoral Psychology* 4 (May 1953): 29-38.

77. For a more complete discussion of Reich's theories see p. 27.

78. Leon Salzman, "A Critique of Wilhelm Reich's Psychoanalytic Theories," *Journal of Pastoral Care* 9 (Autumn 1955): 153-61.

79. Seward Hiltner's Review of *Psychology of Sex Relations* by Theodor Reik, *Pastoral Psychology* 3 (September 1952): 78-80.

80. For a more complete discussion of Reik's theories see Brown, pp. 173-75.

81. Walter Stokes, Review of *Dogma and Compulsion* by Theodor Reik, *Pastoral Psychology* 4 (April 1953): 65-66.

82. Myron C. Madden, "The Crisis of Becoming a Christian," *Pastoral Psychology* 2 (May 1951): 28-31; Paul E. Johnson, "The Lonely Person," *Pastoral Psychology* 8 (June 1957): 41-48; G. Peterson, "Regression in Healing and Salvation," *Pastoral Psychology* 19 (September 1968): 33-39; Paul E. Pfuetze, "The Concept of the Self in Contemporary Psychotherapy," *Pastoral Psychology* 9 (February 1958): 9-19; Seward Hiltner, "Pastoral Psychology and Constructive Theology," *Pastoral Psychology* 4 (June 1953): 17-26.

Chapter Six

1. E. W. Weir, "Summary of a Discussion of Scholastic Psychology and Modern Experimental Psychology," *American Catholic Philosophical Association Proceedings* 12 (December 1936): 109-11.

2. Sister M. Jeannette, "Psychoanalysis," *Catholic School Journal* 31 (April 1931): 130-32.

3. "Cooperation Between Priests and Alienists," *Catholic Charities Review* 33 (January 1939): 14-15.

4. Abridge V. White, "Place of Religion in Psychotherapy," *Catholic World* 162 (October 1945): 80-81.

5. Robert P. Odenwald, "Psychiatry and the Church: No Blanket Condemnation," *Catholic Charities Review* 40 (July 1946): 149-50.

6. Harry McNeill, "Freudians and Catholics," *Commonweal* 46, 1946 pp. 350-53.

7. "Ministering to the Mind," *America*, 2 August 1947. pp. 482-83.

8. C. A. Warwick, "On Casting Out a Devil," *America*, 15 November 1947, pp. 81-82. R. C. Beehan, "Christian Approach to Psychiatry," *Hospital Progress* 29 (April 1948): 29.

9. A. McDonough, "Reliable Psychotherapy," *Sign* 28 (July 1949): 33.

10. William Boyd, "Psychiatrists," *Commonweal*, 7 January 1949, p. 326.

11. See, for example, C. D'Agnostino, "Mental Hygiene and the Clergy," *Catholic Charities Review* 33 (May 1949): 116-19; E. O. Dougherty, "Religion and Psychology," *Catholic Mind* 49 (November 1951): 739-44.

12. See p. 65.

13. Robert P. Odenwald, "Psychiatry and Psychoanalysis," *Sign* 29 (March 1950): 35-36.

14. K. Davies, "What Everyone Should Know About Psychiatry," *Catholic Charities Review* 34 (May 1950): 114-16; Karl Menninger, "Reply," *Commonweal*, 30 May 1952. pp. 200-201.

15. J. Rumaud, "Psychologists vs. Morality," *Cross Currents* 1 (Winter 1951): 26-38.

16. James VanderVeldt cooperated with Robert P. Odenwald to write *Psychiatry and Catholicism* 2nd ed. (New York: Blackstone Division, McGraw Hill, 1958). It was originally published in 1952.

17. James VanderVeldt, "Religion and Mental Health," *Mental Hygiene* 35 (1951): 177-89.

18. Pope Pius XII, "Moral Limits of Medical Research and Treatment," Address to the First International Congress on the Histopathology of the Nervous System, 14 September 1952.

19. The American Catholic Psychological Association was formed in 1950, with the same membership requirements as the American Psychological Association.

20. Karl Stern, "Religion, Philosophy, and Psychiatry," *Guild of Catholic Psychiatrists Bulletin* 1 (December 1952): 18-23.

21. Abridge V. White, "Can Psychologists be Religious?" *Commonweal*, 18 September 1953: 583-84.

22. C. H. de Haas, "Psychology and Religion," *Cross Currents* 4 (Fall 1953): 70-75.

23. Gregory Zilboorg, "The Psychiatrist and the Problem of Religion," *Issues* 2 (December 1954): 5-7.

24. John C. Ford, "May Catholics be Psychoanalyzed?" *Pastoral Psychology* 5 (October 1954): 25-34.

25. Agostino Gemelli, *Psychoanalysis Today* (New York: Kennedy, 1955).

26. Jacques Maritain, "Freudianism and Psychoanalysis," *Cross Currents* 6 (Fall 1956): 307-24.

27. William C. Bier, "Sigmund Freud and the Faith," *America*, 17 November 1956: 192-96.

28. Pope Pius XII, "Morality and Applied Psychology," Address to the Congress of the International Association of Applied Psychology, Rome, 10 April 1958; "On Psychotherapy," Address to the meeting of the International College of Neuro-Psychopharmacology, Rome, 9 September 1958.

29. *Psychiatry and Catholicism*, VanderVeldt and Odenwald, p. 17.

30. Ibid., p. 68-69.

31. Ibid., pp. 99, 102.

32. Ibid., p. 143-48.

33. Ibid., p. 153.

34. Ibid.

35. J. V. Abearonla, "Psychologist Looks at the Problem of Psychology and Ethics," *American Catholic Philosophical Association* 31 (1957): 106-14.

36. Odenwald and VanderVeldt take that position in *Psychiatry and Catholicism*, pp. 345, 304.

37. M. Steck, "Thomistic Psychology and Freud's Psychoanalysis," *Thomist* 21 (April 1958): 25-45.

38. Gregory Zilboorg, "Psychiatry's Moral Sphere," *America*, 3 June 1958: 308-9.

39. Gregory Zilboorg, *Freud and Religion* (Westminster, Maryland: Westminister, 1958).

40. Marc Oraison, "Psychoanalyst and the Confessor," *Cross Currents* 83 (Fall 1958): 63-76.

41. M. Oraison, "Psychoanalysis and Confession," *Commonweal*, 16 January 1959: 424-25.

42. Francis J. Braceland, "A Psychiatrist Examines the Relationship Between Psychiatry and the Catholic Clergy," *Pastoral Psychology* 10 (February 1959): 14-25.

43. Gustave Weigel, "The Challenge of Peace," *Pastoral Psychology* 10 (February 1959): 29-36.

44. Finlan McNamee, "Religion and Psychiatry," *Hospital Progress* 40 (September 1960): 62-65.

45. F. M. Limaco, "Religious Values Must be Acknowledged by Today's Psychologists," *Catholic School Journal* 60 (April 1960): 38-39.

46. John W. Higgins, "Some Considerations of Psychoanalytic Theory," *American Catholic Philosophical Association Proceedings* 35 (1961): 21-44.

47. Alden L. Fisher, "Freud and the Image of Man," *American Catholic Philosophical Association Proceedings* 35 (1961): 45-77.

48. Franz Alexander, "Psychic Determinism and Responsibility," *Bulletin of the Guild of Catholic Psychiatrists* 1 (December 1962): 31-35.

49. P. Sullivan, "Why Catholics Prefer Catholic Psychiatrists," *America*, 9 February 1963. pp. 199-201.

50. Gregory Zilboorg, *Psychoanalysis and Religion* (New York: Farrar, Straus and Cudahy, 1962).

51. Joshua Loth Liebman, *Peace of Mind*, (New York, Simon & Schuster, 1946).

52. A religious book of laws which Jews regard as second in importance only to the Bible.

53. Liebman, p. 19.

54. Sol W. Ginsberg, *Man's Place in God's World: A Psychiatric Evaluation* (Cincinnati: Hebrew Union College–Jewish Institute of Religion, 1948).

55. Joshua A. Fishman, "How Safe is Psychoanalysis?" *Jewish Education* 23 no. 1 (1952): 45-48.

56. Robert L. Katz, "Aspects of Pastoral Psychology and the Rabbinate," *Pastoral Psychology* 5 (October 1954): 35-42.

57. Joseph H. Golnar, "Dilemma of the American Jew," *Jewish Social Service Quarterly* 31 (1954): 165-72.

58. Mortimer Ostow and Ben Ami Scharfstein, *The Need to Believe: The Psychology of Religion* (New York: International University Press, 1954).

59. Abraham N. Franzblau, "The Ministry of Counseling," *Journal of Pastoral Care* 9 (Autumn 1955): 137-44.

60. Louis Linn, "The Need to Believe," in *Judaism and Psychiatry*, ed. Simon Noveck (New York: Basic Books, 1956), pp. 129-34; Louis Linn and Leo M. Schwarz, "The Domains of Psychiatry and Religion," *Pastoral Psychology* 9 (October 1958): 41-49.

61. Noveck, pp. 163-66.

62. Alexander Alan Steinbach, "Psychiatry and Religion Meet," Noveck, p. 1.

63. Abraham N. Franzblau, "Psychiatry and Religion," Noveck, pp. 183-92.

64. Hasidism is a pietistic, ecstatic branch of Judaism, whose members in general retain the characteristic dress and customs of eighteenth-century European Jews.

65. J. H. Gelberman and D. Kobak, "Psychology and Modern Hasidism," *Journal of Pastoral Care* 17 (September 1963): 27-30.

66. Jacob J. Weinstein, "Religion Looks at Psychiatry," *Pastoral Psychology* 9 (November 1958): 25-32.

67. Sandor S. Feldman, "Notes on Some Religious Rites and Ceremonies," *Journal of Hillside Hospital* (1959): 887-92.

68. G. C. Anderson, "Partnership of Theologians and Psychiatrists," *Journal of Religion and Health* 13 (October 1963): 50-69.

69. For the discussion of role of the rabbi, see pp. 71, 130.

Chapter Seven

1. George A. Coe taught a course called "Psychology and Religious Education" at Union Theological Seminary in New York City. He was a pioneer in the field of pre-Freudian psychology of religion.

2. G. A. Coe, "What Constitutes a Scientific Interpretation of Religion?" *Journal of Religion* 6 (May 1926): 225-35.

3. A. E. Hayden, "Spiritual (Religious) Values and Mental Hygiene," *Mental Hygiene* 14 (1930): 779-90.

4. K. R. Stolz, *Pastoral Psychology* (Nashville, Tennessee: Cokesbury Press, 1932).

5. H. C. Link, *The Return to Religion* (New York: Macmillan, 1936).

6. H. N. Wieman, "How Religion Cures Human Ills," *Journal of Religion* 7 (May 1927): 263-76.

7. A. J. Jorden, *A Short Psychology of Religion* (New York: Harpers, 1927).

8. P. B. Herring, *Mind Surgery* (Holyoke, Massachusetts: Elizabeth Thorne Co., 1931).

9. Paul E. Johnson, "Religious Psychology and Health," *Mental Hygiene* 31 (1947): 556-66.

10. E. Steinhal, "Physician and the Minister," *Lutheran Quarterly* 2 (August 1950): 287-96.

11. Editorial, *Journal of Pastoral Psychology* 1 (May 1950): 9-15.

12. Doris Mode, "God-Centered Therapy: A Criticism of Client-Centered Therapy," *Journal of Pastoral Care* 4 (Spring-Summer 1950): 19-23.

13. Anton T. Boisen, "The Period of Beginnings," *Journal of Pastoral Care* 4 (Spring 1951): 13-16.

14. David E. Roberts, "When is Counseling or Psychotherapy Religious?" *Journal of Pastoral Care* 5 (Summer 1952): 15-22.

15. Samuel H. Miller, "Exploring the Boundary between Religion and Psychiatry," *Journal of Pastoral Care* 6 (Summer 1952): 1-18.

16. Joachim Scharfenberg, "The Babylonian Captivity of Pastoral Theology," *Journal of Pastoral Care* 8 (Fall 1954): 125-34. The Rev. Scharfenberg was a minister of the Evangelical (German) Lutheran Church.

17. W. Earl Biddle, "Integration of Religion and Psychiatry," *Pastoral Psychology* 3 (February 1952): 34-41.

18. George O. Evenson, "Reader's Forum," *Pastoral Psychology* 4 (May 1953): 54.

19. Orville S. Walters, "The Minister and the New Counseling," *Journal of Pastoral Care* 7 (Winter 1953): 191-203.

20. A. T. Molligen, "Utilization of Religious Attitudes in Clinical Psychiatry," *Bulletin of the Isaac Ray Medical Library* 2 (1954): 116-35.

21. G. C. Anderson, "Psychiatry's Influence on Religion," *Pastoral Psychology* 7 (September 1956): 745-54.

22. Milton Rosenberg, "The Social Sources of the Current Religious Revival," *Pastoral Psychology* 8 (June 1957): 31-36.

23. Gibson Winter, "Pastoral Counseling or Pastoral Care," *Pastoral Psychology* 8 (February 1957): 16-22.

24. Russell B. Blelzer, "The Minister as a Counselor," *Pastoral Psychology* 8 (March 1957): 28-34.

25. C. Bergendoff, "Mod Imagination and Imago Dei," *Lutheran Quarterly* 10 (May 1958): 99-114.

26. David Elton Trueblood, "The Challenge of Freud," *Pastoral Psychology* 9 (June 1958): 37-44.

27. A. W. Clark, "Toad's Eye View of Psychiatry and Faith," *Journal of Religion and Health* 2 (July 1963): 296-312.

28. Donald F. Krill, "Psychoanalysts, Mowrer and the Existentialists," *Pastoral Psychology* 6 (October 1965): 27-36.

29. Orville S. Walters, "Psychiatrist and Christian Faith," *Christian Century*, 20 July 1960, pp. 47-49.

30. P. Landon, "Psychotherapists and the New Clergy," *Christian Century*, 26 April 1961, pp. 515-56.

31. Orville S. Walters, "Psychiatry-Religion Dialogue," *Christian Century*, 27 December 1961, pp. 1556-58.

32. W. Harden, review of *Crisis in Psychiatry*, by O. Hobart Mowrer, *Christian Century*, 13 September 1961, p. 1080.

33. M. Strendin, "Psychology Without a Soul," *Catholic World* 131 (July 1930): 131-44.

34. C. H. Williamson, "Danger of Psychoanalysis," *Catholic World* 136 (December 1932): 296-301.

35. W. H. Sheldon, "Nature of the Human Mind and Body," *American Catholic Philosophical Association Proceedings* 13 (December 1937): 147-60.

36. W. P. Commins, "What May We Expect of Gestalt Psychology?" *Catholic Educational Review* 35 (March 1937): 135-43.

37. J. A. O'Brien, "Psychiatry and the Confessional," *Ecclesiastical Review* 98 (March 1938): 223-31.

38. W. J. Gerry, "Freud Has Passed and Freudianism Also Goes," *America*, October 1939, pp. 616-17.

39. Rudolf Allers, "Holding up the Mirror of Psychoanalysis," *Catholic Charities Review* 23 (March 1939): 70-72.

40. J. W. Stafford, "Freedom in Experimental Psychology," *American Catholic Philosophical Association Proceedings* 16 (1940): 148-54

41. M. Kant, "Of Cabbages and Cats," *Catholic World* 156 (January 1943): 438-47.

42. "Ministering to the Mind," *America*, 2 August 1947, pp. 482-83.

43. K. Novis, "Cure All: Psychoanalysis," *Catholic World* 167 (June 1948): 218-22.

44. Karl Stern, "Religion and Psychiatry," *Commonweal*, 22 October 1948, pp. 30-33.

45. B. Scheeva, "Religion Marries Psychiatry," *Catholic World* 170 (December 1949): 161-65.

46. A. Stander, "Science behind Psychiatry," *Integrity* 4 (August 1950): 32-38.

47. "Guilt Feelings and Neuroses," *America*, 23 December 1950, p. 350.

48. A. Keenan, "What Can Be Done to a Neurosis," *Integrity* 5 (May 1951): 26-32.

49. D. Dohen, "Unless a Man Be Born Again," *Integrity* 6 (October 1951): 34-40.

50. Pope Pius XII, "Moral Limits of Medical Research and Treatment."

51. G. F. George, "Pope on Psychoanalysis," *America*, 4 October 1952, p. 12.

52. "Pope Pius XII on Psychoanalysis," *America*, 89 2 May 1953, p. 126.

53. J. B. McAllister, "Psychoanalysis and Morality," *New Scholastic* 30 (July 1956): 10-29.

54. J. M. Martin, "Opportunities for the Catholic Psychiatrist," *American Ecclesiastical Review* 135 (August 1956): 37-86.

55. R. B. Nording, "Man's Rationality, a Psychological View," *Catholic Educational Review* 55 (February 1957): 73-81.

56. R. A. De Nardo, "Depth Psychology and the Contribution of Existential Synthesis," *New Scholastic* 32 (April 1958): 187-201.

57. Pope Pius XII, "Morality and Applied Psychology," "On Psychology."

58. M. E. Stock, "Some Moral Issues in Psychoanalysis," *Thomist* 23 (April 1960): 143-88.

Chapter Eight

1. R. R. Willoughby, *A Handbook of Social Psychology* (Worcester, Mass.: Clark University Press, 1935), pp. 461-519.

2. Roger B. Nichols, "Anxiety: An Investigation in Diagnosis and Christian Therapy," *Journal of Pastoral Care* 2 (Winter 1948): 19-26.

3. Rollo May, "Religion and Anxiety," *Pastoral Psychology* 1 (March 1950): 46-49.

4. See pp. 43-44.

5. Rollo May, "Toward an Understanding of Anxiety," *Pastoral Psychology* 1 (March 1950): 25-31.

6. Anton T. Boisen, "The Therapeutic Significance of Anxiety," *Journal of Pastoral Care* 4 (Summer 1951): 1-15.

7. Earl D. Bond, "Anxiety from the Psychiatrist's Viewpoint," *Pastoral Psychology* 2 (March 1951): 14-21.

8. Samuel H. Miller, "Exploring the Boundary between Religion and Psychiatry," *Journal of Pastoral Care* 6 (Summer 1952): 1-11.

9. Isidor Thorner, "Ascetic Protestantism and Alcoholism," *Psychiatry* 16 (1953): 167-76.

10. Review of *The Meaning of Religious Anxiety* by Fred Berthold, *Pastoral Psychology* 7 (February 1956): 50-52.

11. Wayne E. Oates, *Anxiety in the Christian Experience* (Philadelphia: Westminister Press, 1955).

12. Calvin S. Hall, "Freud's Concept of Anxiety," *Pastoral Psychology* 6 (March 1955): 43-48.

13. John Sutherland Bonnell, "Anxiety–The Sickness of Western Civilization," *Pastoral Psychology* 8 (May 1957): 1-14.

14. Seward Hiltner, ed. *Constructive Aspects of Anxiety* (New York: Abingdon Press, 1963) Chapter III.

15. Ibid., Chapter V.

16. Randolf Crump Miller, "Anxiety and Learning," *Pastoral Psychology* 15 (February 1964): 66-75.

17. Odenwald and VanderVeldt, pp. 340-45.

18. Liebman, pp. 90-103.

19. Henry Raphael Gold was a rabbi, a psychoanalyst, and a psychiatrist.

20. Henry Raphael Gold, "Can We Speak of Jewish Neuroses?" in Noveck, pp. 155-60; B. Malzberg, "New Data Relative to the Incidence of Mental Disease Among Jews," *Mental Hygiene* 20 (1936): 80-91; C. Harms, "The Nervous Jew–A Study in Social Psychiatry," *Disorders of the Nervous System* 3 (1942): 47-52.

21. Henry Enoch Kagan, "Fear and Anxiety; A Jewish View," in Noveck, pp. 45-47.

22. John Sutherland Bonnell, "Healing for Mind and Body," *Pastoral Psychology* 1 (March 1950): 30-33.

23. John Sutherland Bonnell, "Religious Disciplines," *Pastoral Psychology* 1 (February 1950); 17-18.

24. Rollo May, "Religion, Psychotherapy, and the Achievement of Selfhood," *Pastoral Psychology* 2 (November 1951): 15-20.

25. J. Hoffman, "Psychological, Pathological Guilt Feelings and Psychiatry," *Journal of Pastoral Care* 6 no. 2 (1952): 42-52.

26. Erich Lindeman, "Symptomatology and Management of Acute Grief," *Pastoral Psychology* 14 (September 1963): 8-18.

27. Adolph Koberle, "The Problem of Guilt," trans. John W. Duberstein, *Pastoral Psychology* 8 (December 1957): 33-39.

28. Le Roy Alden, "Distortions of a Sense of Guilt," *Pastoral Psychology* 15 (February 1964): 16-26.

29. Leon M. Salzman, "Guilt, Responsibility, and the Unconscious," *Pastoral Psychology* 15 (November 1964): 17-26.

30. Odenwald and VanderVeldt, pp. 340-44.

31. Liebman, pp. 30-33.

32. Alexander Alan Steinbach, "Depression: A Jewish View," in Noveck, pp. 72-83.

33. David Kairys, "Conscience and Guilt: A Psychiatric View," Noveck, pp. 13-23.

34. Edward T. Sandrow, "Conscience and Guilt: A Jewish View," Noveck, pp. 24-31.

35. Simon P. Noveck, "Editor's Note," Noveck, p. 116.

36. C. E. Barbour, *Sin and the New Psychology* (New York: Abingdon Press, 1930).

37. Ralph Higgins, "Client-Centered Psychotherapy and Christian Doctrine," *Journal of Pastoral Care* 3 (Spring 1949): 1-12.

38. Edith H. Weigert, "Psychiatry and Sin," *Journal of Pastoral Care* 4 no. 1-2 (1950): 43-49.

39. Ernest E. Bruder, "Psychotherapy and Some of Its Theological Implications," *Journal of Pastoral Care* 6 (Summer 1952): 28.

40. O. Hobart Mowrer, "Transference and Scrupulosity," (reprint) *Journal of Religion and Health* 23 (July 1963): 3-43.

41. Wayne E. Oates, Review of *Protestant Pastoral Counseling* by O. H. Mowrer, *Christian Century*, 3 April 1963, pp. 430-31.

42. James A. Knight, "The Use and Misuses of Religion by the Emotionally Disturbed," *Pastoral Psychology* 13 (March 1962): 8-10.

43. Vincent Mahoney, "Scrupulosity from the Psychoanalytic Viewpoint," *The Guild of Catholic Psychiatrists Bulletin* 2 (December 1957): 11-21.

44. Odenwald and VanderVeldt, pp. 380-89.

45. Henry Enoch Kagan, "Fear and Anxiety: A Jewish View," in Noveck, pp. 52.

46. Edward T. Sandrow, "Conscience and Guilt: A Jewish View," Noveck, pp. 24-31.

47. Sigmund Freud, *Mourning and Melancholia.*

48. William F. Rogers, "Needs of the Bereaved," *Pastoral Psychology* 1 (July 1950): 17-21.

49. "The Consultation Clinic, The Pastor and Suicide," *Pastoral Psychology* 4 (December 1953): 51-54.

50. Erich Lindeman, "Symptomatology and Management of Acute Grief," *Pastoral Psychology* 14 (September 1963): 8-18.

51. Hattie Rosenthal, "Psychotherapy for the Dying," *Pastoral Psychology* 14 (June 1963): 50-56.

52. William F. Rogers, "The Pastor's Work with Grief," *Pastoral Psychology* 14 (September 1963): 19-26.

53. Liebman, p. 113-23.

54. Simon Noveck, "A Jewish View of Grief," in Noveck, pp. 105-12.

55. Jack D. Spiro, *A Time to Mourn: The Dynamics of Mourning in Judaism* (Cincinnati, Hebrew Union College-Jewish Institute of Religion, 1961).

56. Edith Weigert, "Love and Fear: a Psychiatric Interpretation," *Journal of Pastoral Care* 5 (Summer 1951): 12-22.

57. Paul E. Johnson,"Christian Love and Self Love," *Pastoral Psychology* 2 (March 1951): 14-20.

58. Paul E. Johnson, "Contributions of Psychology to the Teacher of Religion," *Journal of Bible and Religion* 24 (July 1956): 167-72.

59. Odenwald and VanderVeldt, p. 127.

60. Ruth Levy, "The Implications of Psychiatry for Religion," *Reconstructionist* 16 (1951): 26-29.

61. Paul E. Johnson, "Jesus as a Practicing Psychologist: Jesus was a Physician of Souls," *Pastoral Psychology* 2 (December 1951): 17-21. The same position was taken by William E. Hulme, *Counseling and Theology* (Philadelphia: Muhlenberg, 1956).

62. John Dolard and Neale E. Miller, "Free Association Without Understanding the Past," *Pastoral Psychology* 3 (February 1952): 31-34.

63. Donald S. Arbuckle, "Therapy is for All," *Journal of Pastoral Care* 6 (Winter 1952): 34-39.

64. Aleck Dodd, "Relationship Therapy as Religion," *Journal of Psychotherapy and Religion, Proceedings* 1 (1954): 41-51.

65. Liebman.

66. Wilfred Daim, "On Depth-Psychology and Salvation," *Journal of Psychotherapy and Religion, Proceedings* 2 (1952): 24-37.

67. Anton T. Boisen, "Economic Distress and Religious Experience: A Study of the Holy Rollers," *Psychiatry* 2 (1939): 185-94.

68. Anton T. Boisen, "The Genesis and Significance of Mystical Identification in Cases of Mental Disorders," *Psychiatry* 15 (1952): 287-96.

69. D. H. Salman, "The Psychology of Religious Experience," *R. M. Bucke Memorial Society for the Study of Religious Experience: Proceedings of the First Annual Conference* (Montreal, Canada, np.): 85-111.

70. Alfred B. Haas, "The Therapeutic Value of Hymns," *Pastoral Psychology* 1 (December 1950): 39-42.

71. James H. Burns, "The Application of Psychology to Preaching," *Pastoral Psychology* 3 (March 1952): 29-33.

72. Earl H. Furgeson, "Preaching and Personality," *Pastoral Psychology* 10 (October 1959): 9-14.

73. Luther E. Woodward, "Contributions of the Minister to Mental Hygiene," *Pastoral Psychology* 1 (February 1950): 19-25; (May 1950): 43-47.

74. Anton T. Boisen, "Psychiatric Approach to the Study of Religion," *Journal of Religious Education* 23 (March 1928): 201-7.

75. Anton T. Boisen, *The Exploration of the Inner World: A Study of Mental Disorder and Religious Experience* (Chicago: Willett, Clark, 1936).

76. Anton T. Boisen, "Problem of Sin and Salvation in the Light of Psychopathology," *Journal of Religion* and Health 22 (July 1942): 288-301.

77. Harry M. Tiebout, "The Act of Surrender in the Treatment of the Alcoholic," *Pastoral Psychology* 1 (May 1950): 42-50.

78. William S. Hill, "The Psychology of Conversion," *Pastoral Psychology* 6 (November 1955): 43-63.

79. Carl Christensen, "Religious Conversion in Adolescence," *Pastoral Psychology* 16 (September 1965): 17-36.

80. Anton T. Boisen, "Ideas of Prophetic Mission," *Journal of Pastoral Care* 12 (Spring 1961): xvi-6.

81. Harry M. Tiebout, "Alcoholics Anonymous: An Experiment of Nature," *Pastoral Psychology* 13 (April 1962): 45-62.

82. Earl H. Furgeson, "The Definition of Religious Conversion," *Pastoral Psychology* 16 (September 1965): 8-16.

83. Milton R. Saperstein, "The Meaning of Personal Religious Experience," Noveck, pp. 119-24.

84. D. Yellowless, *Psychology's Defense of the Faith* (New York: R. R. Smith, 1930).

85. J. R. Oliver, *Pastoral Psychiatry and Mental Health* (New York: Scribner, 1932).

86. Anton T. Boisen, "The Problem of Sin and Salvation in the Light of Psychology," *Journal of Religion and Health* 22 (July 1942): 288-301.

87. Sylvanus M. Duvall, "Sex Morals in the Context of Religion," *Pastoral Psychology* 3 (May 1952): 33-37.

88. Joseph Fletcher, "A Moral Philosophy of Sex," *Pastoral Psychology* 4 (February 1953): 31-37.

89. Ashley Montagu, "The Origins of Love and Hate," *Pastoral Psychology* 4 (December 1953): 46-48.

90. Alfred C. Kinsey, *Sexual Behavior in the Human Male* (Philadelphia: W. B. Saunders Co., 1948); *Sexual Behavior in the Human Female* (Philadelphia: W. B. Saunders Co., 1953).

91. Karl Menninger, "Kinsey's Study of Sexual Behavior in the Human Male and Female," *Pastoral Psychology* 5 (February 1954): 43-85.

92. Gothard Booth, "Masturbation," *Pastoral Psychology* 5 (November 1954): 13-20.

93. Freud said that the passionate feeling he had felt towards his wife dissipated after a few years of marriage.

94. William Graham Cole, *Sex and Christianity* (New York: Oxford University Press, 1955).

95. Adolf Meyer, "Repression, Freedom and Discipline," *Pastoral Psychology* 7 (September 1956): 13-18.

96. Lester Kirkendull, "Premarital Sex Relations; The Problem and its Implications," *Pastoral Psychology* 7 (April 1956): 46-56.

97. Norman C. Morgan, "Religion in Psychotherapy," *Pastoral Psychology* 8 (October 1957): 17-22.

98. Vere V. Loper, "A Christian Tries to Hold Homes Together," *Pastoral Psychology* 8 (December 1957): 9-14.

99. D. C. McClelland, "Religious Overtones in Psychoanalysis," *Theology Today* 16 (April 1959): 40-64.

100. Milton J. Huber, "Counseling the Single Woman," *Pastoral Psychology* 10 (April 1959): 11-18.

101. Carroll A. Wise, "Education of the Pastor for Marriage Counseling," *Pastoral Psychology* 10 (December 1959): 15-18.

102. Thomas J. Bingham, "Pastoral Ethical Notes on Problems of Masturbation," *Pastoral Psychology* 11 (June 1960): 19-23.

103. "Consultation Clinic – Masturbation," *Pastoral Psychology* 11 (May 1961): 51-57.

104. Odenwald and VanderVeldt, p. 440.

105. Ibid., pp. 450-57.

106. Ibid., pp. 408-13.

107. Ibid., pp. 430-33.

Chapter Nine

1. Francis L. Strickland, "Pastoral Psychology – A Retrospect," *Pastoral Psychology* 4 (October 1953): 9-12.

2. "Pastoral Psychology Retrospect," Editorial, *Pastoral Psychology* 4 (October 1953): 15.

3. "Origins of Clinical Pastoral Training," *Pastoral Psychology* 4 (October 1953): 13-15.

4. Fred Eastman, "Father of the Clinical Pastoral Movement," *Journal of Pastoral Care* 7 (Spring 1953): 3-7.

5. Ibid.

6. Ibid.

7. Boisen and Guiles agreed that seeing the final stages of mental disorder could shed light on earlier stages.

8. Frederick C. Kuether, "The Council for Clinical Training," *Pastoral Psychology* 4 (October 1953): 17-20.

9. James H. Burns, "The Institute for Pastoral Care," *Pastoral Psychology* 4 (October 1953): 21-24.

10. Ernest E. Bruder, "Clinical Pastoral Training as a Hospital Medium in Public Relations," *Pastoral Psychology* 4 (November 1953): 27-36.

11. Ernest E. Bruder and Marian L. Barb, "A Survey of 10 Years of Clinical Pastoral Training at St. Elizabeth's Hospital," *Journal of Pastoral Care* 10 (Summer 1956): 86-94.

12. Anton T. Boisen, "The Minister as Counselor," *Journal of Pastoral Care* 2 (Spring 1948): 13-22.

13. Seward Hiltner, "The American Association of Pastoral Counselors: A Critique," *Pastoral Psychology* 15 (April 1964): 8-16.

14. Howard J. Clinebell, "The Challenge of the Specialty of Pastoral Counseling," *Pastoral Psychology* 15 (April 1964): 17-28.

15. Ibid. A report to the Methodist Interboard Consultation on Pastoral Counseling Centers, given April 5, 1963 at Boston University, said that 80% of counseling centers had developed since 1955 and that 50% had developed since 1960.

16. The Metropolitan Church Federation in St. Louis, Missouri, treated 200 families, mostly for marital problems, and considered that the treatment was helpful in 110 cases, according to Robert Deitchman, "The Evolution of a Ministerial Counseling Center," *Journal of Pastoral Care* 11 (Winter 1957): 7-14. Other clinical training programs existed, such as the Lutheran Institute of Pastoral Care at Milwaukee Hospital, and programs run by the friends of clinical training.

17. By 1956 almost half of the theological seminaries in the United States offered ten or more courses in psychology. E. Llewellyn Queener, "The Psychological Training of Ministers," *Pastoral Psychology* 7 (October 1956): 29-34.

18. Robert C. Dodds, "A Parochial Evaluation of Clinical Pastoral Training," *Journal of Pastoral Care* 2 (Fall 1948): 22-25.

19. Wayne E. Oates, "Role of Religion in Psychoses," *Journal of Pastoral Care* 3 (Spring 1949): 21-35; "Pastoral Psychology in the South," *Pastoral Psychology* 2 (May 1951): 9-10.

20. Russell C. Dicks, *Pastoral Work and Personal Counseling*, rev. ed. (New York: Macmillan Co., 1949).

21. John Rea Thomas, "Evaluation of Clinical Pastoral Training and 'Part Time' Training in a General Hospital," *Journal of Pastoral Care* 12 (Spring 1958): 28-34.

22. Kim Edward Lester, "A Critical Study of Selective Changes in Protestant Theological Students with Clinical Pastoral Education," in "Report on Doctoral Dissertations," *Pastoral Psychology* 13 (March 1962): 39-40.

23. Berkley Hawthorne, *A Critical Analysis of Protestant Church Counseling Centers* (Boston, Massachusetts: Boston University, 1960).

24. Cajetan Cambell, "An Evaluation of Catholic Chaplains' Training," *Guild of Catholic Psychiatrists Bulletin* 6 no. 2, (April 1959): 19-21.

25. Finlan McNamee, "Religion and Psychiatry," *Hospital Progress* 40 (September 1960): 62-65.

26. Robert L. Katz, "Aspects of Pastoral Psychology and the Rabbinate," *Pastoral Psychology* 5 (October 1954): 35-42.

27. Noveck, p. 193.

28. H. F. Dunbar, "Mental Hygiene and Religious Teaching," *Mental Hygiene* 19 (1935): 535-37.

29. M. E. Kirkpatrick, "Mental Hygiene and Religion," *Mental Hygiene* 24 (1940): 378-89.

30. William C. Menninger, "Psychiatry and Religion," *Pastoral Psychology* 1 (February 1950): 14-16.

31. "Consultation Clinic: How far can a pastor go with an extreme neurotic?" *Pastoral Psychology* 2 (January 1952): 49-55.

32. Charles F. Brooks, "Some Limiting Factors in Pastoral Counseling," *Pastoral Psychology* 2 (March 1951): 26-31.

33. Thomas J. Bingham, "The Religious Element in Marriage Counseling," *Pastoral Psychology* 2 (May 1951): 14-18.

34. Anton T. Boisen, "The Distinctive Task of the Minister," *Pastoral Psychology* 3 (April 1952): 10-15.

35. Karl Menninger, "The Character of the Therapist," *Pastoral Psychology* 9 (November 1958): 14-18.

36. John Sutherland Bonnell, "The Practice of Counseling in the Local Church," *Pastoral Psychology* 11 (February 1960): 24-30.

37. A. Mansell Pattison, "Functions of the Clergy in the Community Mental Health Centers," *Pastoral Psychology* 16 (May 1965): 21-26.

38. For a discussion of Carl Rogers and Existentialist Psychotherapy see pp. 49-54.

39. Wayne E. Oates, "Levels of Pastoral Care: The New Testament Concept of a Health-Giving Ministry," *Pastoral Psychology* 2 (May 1951): 11-16.

40. Seward Hiltner, *The Christian Shepherd* (New York: Abingdon Press, 1959).

41. Seward Hiltner and Lowell Colston, *The Context of Pastoral Counseling* (New York: Abingdon Press, 1961).

42. Glenn V. Ramsey, "Aids for the Minister in Detecting Early Maladjustment," *Pastoral Psychology* 14 (February 1963): 41-51.

43. Rudolf Allers, "Impediments of the Human Act," *Ecclesiastical Review* 100 (March 1937): 208-16.

44. Charles A. Currian, "A Catholic Psychologist Looks at Pastoral Counseling," *Pastoral Psychology* 10 (February 1959): 21-28.

45. Odenwald and VanderVeldt, pp. 237-49.

46. Charles Miller, "The Significance for the Center of Community Organization in Metropolitan Communities," *Jewish Social Service Quarterly* 27 (1950): 53-61.

47. Abraham Franzblau, "Psychiatry and Religion," in Noveck, p. 193.

48. Yeshiva University is an Orthodox university which tries to combine religious orthodoxy with knowledge of the modern world.

49. I. Fred Hollander, "The Specific Nature of the Clergy's Role in Mental Health," *Pastoral Psychology* 10 (November 1959): 11-22.

50. Enoch Kagan, "The Role of the Rabbi as Counselor," *Pastoral Psychology* 5 (October 1954): 17-23.

51. Enoch Kagan, "The Rabbi and the Community," *Journal of Religion and Health* 13 (July 1950): 50-61.

52. Noveck, p. 190.

53. Kagan, "The Rabbi and the Community."

54. Jeshaia Schnitzer, "Rabbis and Counseling," *Jewish Social Studies* 20 (1958): 131-52.

55. Don C. Shaw, "Some General Considerations on the Religious Care of the Mentally Ill," *Journal of Clinical Pastoral Work* 1 no. 2 (1947): 20-25.

56. Ernest Bruder, "A Clinically Trained Religious Ministry in the Mental Hospital," *Quarterly Review of Psychiatry and Neurology* 2 (1947): 543-52.

57. Anton T. Boisen, "The Service of Worship in a Mental Hospital: Its Therapeutic Significance," *Journal of Clinical Pastoral Work* 2 no. 1 (1948): 19-25.

58. William R. Andrew, "Faith and Pastoral Counseling," *Journal of Clinical Pastoral Work* 3 no. 2 (1949): 61-82.

59. Russell C. Dicks, "The Hospital Chaplain," *Pastoral Psychology* 1 (March 1950): 50-54.

60. Robert M. Gluckman, "The Chaplain as a Member of the Diagnostic Clinical Team," *Journal of Pastoral Care* 8 (Spring 1954): 83-87.

61. Calvin Hall, "The Function of the Psychiatric Chaplain," *Journal of Pastoral Care* 9 (August 1955): 145-52.

62. I. M. Melamed, "The Jewish Prisoner," *Jewish Social Service Quarterly* 31 (1954): 173-79.

63. Robert V. Seliger, "Religious and Similar Experiences and Revelations in Patients with Alcohol Problems," *Journal of Clinical Psychotherapy* 7-8 (1947): 728-31.

64. Howard J. Clinebell, "American Protestantism and the Problem of Alcoholism," *Journal of Pastoral Work* 3 no. 1 (1949): 199-215.

65. Joan K. Jackson, "Alcoholism as a Family Crisis," *Pastoral Psychology* 13 (April 1962): 8-18.

66. E. A. Verdery, "Pastoral Care of the Alcoholic's Family After Sobriety," *Pastoral Psychology* 13 (April 1962): 30-38.

67. Howard J. Clinebell, "Pastoral Care of the Alcoholic's Family Before Sobriety," *Pastoral Psychology* 13 (April 1962): 19-29.

68. Alfred A. Gross, "The Homosexual in Society," *Pastoral Psychology* 1 (March 1950): 38-48.

69. Aaron L. Rutledge, "Concepts of God among the Emotionally Upset," *Pastoral Psychology* 2 (May 1951): 22-25.

70. Edmund Bergler, "Homosexuality: Disease or Way of Life," *Pastoral Psychology* 8 (June 1957): 49-52.

71. Hubert Hendin, "What a Pastor Ought to Know about Suicide," *Pastoral Psychology* 4 (December 1953): 4-5.

72. F. C. Cesarman, "The Conversion of Sex Offenders During Psychotherapy: Two Cases," *Journal of Pastoral Care* 11 (February 1957): 25-35.

73. Judson D. Howard, "Churches and Mental Illness," *Pastoral Psychology* 4 (October 1953): 35-38.

74. John Sutherland Bonnell, "Counseling Divorced Persons," *Pastoral Psychology* 9 (June 1958): 11-15.

75. Charles William Stewart, "Divorce Shatters One's World View and Makes One Question Life's Meaning," *Pastoral Psychology* 14 (April 1963): 10-16.

76. Special issue on *The Church and Mental Retardation, Pastoral Psychology* 13 (September 1962).

77. Milton I. Levine and Reuel L. Howe, "Pediatrics and the Church: A Symposium" *Journal of Pastoral Care* 3 (Fall-Winter 1949): 39-44.

78. Stuart McIntyre Finch, "The Pastor's Role with the Anxious Child," *Pastoral Psychology* 2 (October 1951): 23-28.

79. Samuel Southard, "The Evangelism of Children," *Pastoral Psychology* 7 (December 1956): 31-37.

80. Earl Loomis, "Child Psychiatry and Religion," *Pastoral Psychology* 7 (September 1956): 27-33.

81. Phillip Polatin, "Children and Divorce," *Pastoral Psychology* 9 (October 1958): 33-40.

82. John H. Snow, "Understanding 'Troublesome' Behavior in Children," *Journal of Pastoral Care* 13 (Spring 1959): 1-12.

83. Earl H. Furgeson, "Preaching and Counseling Functions of the Minister," *Journal of Pastoral Care* 2 (Winter 1948): 11-18.

84. Seward Hiltner, *Pastoral Counseling* (Nashville, Tennessee: Abingdon Cokesbury Press, 1949).

85. Ralph Higgins, "Client-Centered Psychotherapy and Christian Doctrine," *Journal of Pastoral Care* 3 (Spring 1949): 1-12.

86. Wayne E. Oates, "The Role of Religion in the Psychoses," *Journal of Pastoral Care* 3 (Spring 1949): 21-30.

87. Russell C. Dicks, "Sacrament of Conversation," *Pastoral Psychology* 2 (May 1951): 17-21.

88. Howard J. Clinebell, "Ego Psychology and Pastoral Counseling," *Pastoral Psychology* 14 (February 1963): 26-36.

89. A. B. Bioren, "Theory of Perception in Rogerian Therapy," *Catholic Educational Review* 60 (January 1962): 62.

90. Odenwald and VanderVeldt, p. 277.

91. Charles A. Currian, "The Counseling Relationship," *Journal of Counseling Psychology* 6 (1959): 266-70: "Religious Factors and Values in Counseling," *Catholic Counselor* 3 (1958): 3-5, 24.

92. William C. Bier, "Goals in Pastoral Counseling," *Pastoral Psychology* 10 (February 1959): 7-13.

93. Peter P. Girende and Nathaniel J. Paollome, "Client Rapport and the Counselor's Religious Status: An Exploration," *Journal National Conference of Catholic Guidance Counselors* 9 no.4 (1965): 208-19.

94. Harry J. Brevis, "Counseling Prison Inmates," *Pastoral Psychology* 7 (February 1956): 35-42.

95. Jeshaia Schnitzer, "Rabbis and Counseling," *Jewish Social Studies* 20 (1958): 131-52.

96. Robert C. Leslie, "Group Therapy: A New Approach for the Church," *Journal of Pastoral Care* 5 (Spring 1951): 36-45.

97. Clifton E. Kew and Clinton J. Kew, "Principles and Values of Group Psychotherapy under Church Auspices," *Pastoral Psychology* 6 (April 1955): 37-48.

98. Clifton E. Kew, "Group Psychotherapy in a Church Setting," *Pastoral Psychology* 1 (January 1951): 31-37.

99. Rollin J. Fairbanks, "Cooperation Between Clergy and Psychiatrists," *Pastoral Psychology* 2 (September 1951): 19-23.

100. C. W. Hyde and Robert C. Leslie, "Introduction to Group Therapy for Graduate Students," *Journal of Pastoral Care* 6 no.2 (1952): 19-27.

101. Anton T. Boisen, "Group Therapy: The Elgin Plan," *Pastoral Psychology* 5 (March 1954): 33-38.

102. Clifton E. Kew, "Group Healing in the Church," *Pastoral Psychology* 5 (March 1954): 44-50.

103. Robert C. Leslie, "Group Therapy: A New Approach for the Church," *Journal of Pastoral Care* 5 (Spring 1951):36-45.

104. Robert C. Leslie, "Pastoral Group Therapy," *Journal of Pastoral Care* 6 no. 2 (1952): 56-61.

105. "Consultation Clinic," *Pastoral Psychology* 5 (April 1954): 57-58.

106. N. C. Peterson and Beverly Farms, "Group Dynamics Found in Scriptures," *Group Psychotherapy* 15 no. 2 (1962): 126-28.

107. Alvin S. Bobroff, "Religious Psychodrama," *Group Psychotherapy* 16 (1963): 36-38.

108. Herbert Hold and Charles Wenich, "Group Pastoral Counseling," *Pastoral Psychology* 14 (November 1963): 13-22.

109. Ernest E. Bruder, "Clinical Pastoral Training as a Hospital Medium in Public Relations," *Pastoral Psychology* 4 (November 1953): 27-36.

110. Roy A. Burkhart, "Minister's Own Freedom," *Pastoral Psychology* 1(March 1950): 10-12.

111. Blanche Carrier, "Counseling Pre-Ministerial Students," *Pastoral Psychology* 2 (November 1951): 21-25.

112. Carl W. Christensen, "Role of the Psychiatrist Consultant to a Seminary," *Journal of Pastoral Care* 9 (Spring 1955): 1-7.

113. Daniel Blain, "Fostering the Mental Health of Ministers," *Pastoral Psychology* 9 (March 1958): 9-18.

114. M. O. Williams, "The Psychological-Psychiatric Appraisal of Candidates for Missionary Service," *Pastoral Psychology* 9 (December 1958): 41-44.

115. Carroll A. Wise, "The Call to the Ministry," *Pastoral Psychology* 9 (December 1958): 9-17.

116. Margaretta K. Bowers, *Conflicts of the Clergy* (New York: Thomas Nelson & Sons, 1963).

117. H. B. Schoelfield, "Psychoanalysis and the Parish Ministry," Address, *Journal of Religion and Health* 2 (January 1963): 112-28.

118. By 1965, the Rabbinical Seminary of America, an Orthodox seminary at 69th Avenue and Kessel Street, Forest Hills, New York, was offering courses in clinical psychology and field work in pastoral counseling.

119. Gothard Booth, "Basic Concepts of Psychosomatic Medicine," *Pastoral Psychology* 2 (October 1951): 11-18.

120. Odenwald and VanderVeldt, pp. 56-71.

121. Liebman, pp. 34, 91.

122. Gold, in Noveck, pp. 155-60.

123. C. Cooper, *Seven Psychological Portraits: A Handbook for Parents and Teachers* (Milwaukee: Morehouse, 1928).

124. A. J. Meyers, "Use of Fear in Religious Education," *Religious Education* 18 (1923): 908-13.

125. V. E. Marriott, "New Flowers of the Spirit," *Religious Education* 24 (1929): 250-62.

126. B. S. Winchester, *The Church and Adult Education* (New York: R. R. Smith, 1930).

127. J. A. Charters, "The Opportunity of the Church for Sex Education," *Religious Education* 27 (1932): 428-34.

128. S. C. Fahs, "How Childish Should a Child's Religion Be," *Religious Education* 24 (1929): 910-17.

129. J. W. Andrus, "Traits and Characteristics of Young Children," *Religious Education* 24 (1929): 927-29.

130. C. G. McCormick, "The Emotions and a Positive Morality," *Religious Education* 42 (1947): 271-74.

131. William B. Terhune, "Religion and Psychiatry," *Journal of Pastoral Care* 2 no. 2 (1948): 15-21.

132. Ernest M. Ligon, "Possible Contributions of Recent Researchers in Psychology to Religious Education," *Religious Education* 44 (1949): 211-16

133. Roy A. Burkhart, "The Church Program of Education in Marriage and the Family: From Birth to Twelve," *Pastoral Psychology* 2 (November 1951): 10-14.

134. Walter Houston Clark, "The Psychology of Religion and the Understanding of Man in Religious Education," *Religious Education* 54 (1959): 18-23.

135. Stuart M. Finch and Edwin H. Kroor, "Some Educational Factors in the Religious Education of Children," *Religious Education* 54 (1959): 36-43.

136. Richard P. Vaughn, "Counseling the Former Nun," *National Catholic Guidance Counselors Journal* 9 (Winter 1965): 93-101; A. Summo, "The Counselor and Individual Psychological Testing," *Catholic Counselor* 5 (Fall 1960): 1-3; W. Angers, "Guidelines for Counselors for MMPI Interpretation," *Catholic Counselor* 7 (Spring 1963): 120-24.

137. "Full Time Psychologist, An Experiment," *Catholic School Journal* 39 (February 1939): 41-43.

138. M. Carelton, "Pre-Registration Guidance in Catholic Colleges," *Catholic Educational Review* 40 (1942): 162-68.

139. James F. Moynihan, "Student Counseling in Catholic Education," *Higher Education* 18 (1947): 154-58; E. A. Leonard, "Counseling in the Catholic High Schools of the Middle Western States," *Catholic Educational Review* 44 (1946): 483-91.

140. Robert E. Doyle, "Guidance Services in Metropolitan Catholic Schools: A Status Report," *National Catholic Guidance Conference Journal* 9 no. 4 (1965): 227-29.

141. J. W. Stafford, "Undergraduate Preparation for Clinical Psychology," bibliog., *Catholic Educational Review* 47 (February 1949): 83-91; Walter Wilkens, "Another Viewpoint on the Psychology of Personality Development," *Hospital Progress* 31 (October 1950): 314-46; T. J. Cannon, "Function of Psychology Courses in a Catholic College," *Catholic Educational Review* 51 (November 1953): 596-603; "High School Curriculum Should Include Psychology," *Catholic Educational Review* 51 (January 1953): 52; W. A. Kelly, "Preparation of the Instructor in Educational Psychology," *Catholic Educational Review* 52 (February 1954): 102-12.

142. Simon P. Noveck, "Editor's Note," in Noveck, p. 117; Hector J. Ritley, "The Value of Religious Education," Ibid., pp. 143-53.

143. Boris M. Levinson, "The Intelligence of Applicants for Admission to Jewish Day Schools," *Jewish Sociological Studies* 19 (1957): 129-40.

144. The testing considered in this chapter was done almost exclusively by or for religious groups. When the testing was reported in journals of psychology, it will be assumed that testing was done to further academic interests in that field and did not necessarily represent a concern of religious workers.

145. H. Hartshorne, M. May, et al., "Testing the Knowledge of Right and Wrong," *Religious Education Monograph* 9 no. 1 (1927): 72; Ernest M. Ligon, :"A Plea for the Child," *Presbyterian Tribute* 23 (January 1934): 51.

146. P. R. Stevic, "A Study in Feeling of Conformity in Religion," *Religious Education* 28 (1933): 364-47; M. C. Smith and J.E. Barthurst, "Tests and Measurement in Religious Education," *Religious Education* 27 (1932): 439-42; R. G. Bose,

"Religious Concepts of Children," *Religious Education* 24 (1929): 24; R. Bain, "Religious Attitudes of College Students," *American Journal of Sociology* 32 (1927): 766-70. This study tested the same attitudes tested by Leuba in 1917; E. T. Clark, *The Psychology of Religious Awakening* (New York: MacMillan, 1929).

147. Emma Pixley and Emma Beekman, "City Schools: The Faith of Youth as Shown by a Survey in Public Schools of Los Angeles," *Religious Education* 44 (1949): 336-42; A. D. Woodruff, "Students' Verbalized Values," *Religious Education* 38 (1943): 321-24; Walter R. Harrison, "A Study of Church Attitudes in the East Baton Rouge Area," *Religious Education* 47 (1952): 39-52.

148. Philip M. Smith, "Prisoners' Attitudes Toward Organized Religion," *Religious Education* 51 (1956): 462-64; Oliver E. Graebner, "Children's Concepts of God," *Inter-Institutional Seminar in Child Development, Collected Papers* (1957), pp. 184-92.

149. "Consultation Clinic," *Pastoral Psychology* 2 (September 1951): 41-51; David R. Mace, "The Minister's Role in Marriage Preparation," *Pastoral Psychology* 3 (May 1952): 45-48; George H. Weger and Charles V. Gerkin, "A Religious Story Test; Some Findings with Delinquent Boys," *Journal of Pastoral Care* 7 no. 2 (1952): 77-90; Roy A. Burkhart, "A Program of Pre-Marital Counseling," *Pastoral Psychology* 1 (September 1950): 25-34.

150. John C. Whitcomb, "The Relationship of Personality Characteristics of Ministers to Adjustment," *Religious Education* 52 (1957): 371-74; Frederick Kling, "A Study of Testing as Related to the Ministry," *Religious Education* 53 (1958): 243-48; Gothard Booth, "Unconscious Motivation in the Choice of the Ministry," *Pastoral Psychology* 9 (August 1958): 18-24.

151. Jules H. Masserman and Ralph T. Palmer, "Psychiatric and Psychological Tests for Ministerial Personnel," *Pastoral Psychology* 12 (March 1961): 24-31; Frederick Kling, "Value Structures and the Minister's Purpose," *Pastoral Psychology* 12 (March 1961): 13-23; G. E. Whitlock, "Choice of the Ministry as an Active or Passive Decision," *Pastoral Psychology* 12 (March 1962): 31-45; G. E. Whitlock, "Role and Self-Concepts in the Choice of the Ministry as a Vocation," *Journal of Pastoral Care* 17 (Winter 1963): 208-17.

152. John Richard Fowler, "What the Pastor Should Know about Psychological Tests," *Pastoral Psychology* 15 (March 1964): 24-29.

153. Orlo Strunk and Kenneth E. Reed, "The Learning of Empathy," *Journal of Pastoral Care* 14 (Spring 1960): 44-48.

154. John Kasa Schommer, "Participation, Religious Knowledge and Scholastic Aptitude," *Journal for the Scientific Study of Religion* 1 (1961): 88-97; Howard L. Parsons, "Students at Six Colleges and Universities," *Religious Education* 58 no. 6 (1963): 538-44; Andrew M. Greeley, "A Note on the Origins of Religious Differences," *Journal for the Scientific Study of Religion* 3 (1963): 321-31.

155. Stanley Gordon, "Personality and Attitude Correlates of Religious Conversion," *Journal for the Scientific Study of Religion* 4 no. 10 (1964): 60-63; P. Kildahl, "The Personalities of Sudden Religious Converts," *Pastoral Psychology* 16

(September 1965): 37-44; Ewing C. Cooley and Jerry B. Hutton, "Adolescent Religious Response to Religious Appeal as Related to IPAT Anxiety," *Journal of Social Psychology* 67 no. 2 (1965): 325-27.

156.   M. Richard Peters, "Study of the Intercorrelations of Personality Traits Among a Group of Novices in Religious Communities," *Catholic Educational Review* 47 (January 1949): 40; Henry R. Burke, *Personality Traits of Successful Minor Seminarians* (Washington, D. C.: Catholic University Press, 1947); Brian Lhota, *Vocational Interests of Catholic Priests* in *Studies in Psychology and Psychiatry*, (Washington, D. C.: Catholic University Press, 1948).

157.   Joseph Kurich, "Psychiatric and Psychological Selection of Candidates for the Sisterhood," *Guild of Catholic Psychiatrists Bulletin* 1 (1960): 19-25; W. J. Kennedy, "Psychiatric Tests for Seminarians," *National Catholic Education Association Bulletin* 51 (August 1954): 89-95; W. C. Bier, "Psychological Tests in the Screening of Candidates in the Minor Seminary," *National Catholic Educational Association Bulletin* 51 (August 1954): 128-35; John B. Murray, "Personality Study of Priests and Seminarians," *Homiletic and Pastoral Review* 49 (1958): 443-47; Richard P. Vaughn, "The Neurotic Religious," *Review of Religious* 17 (1958): 271-78; "Notes and News," *Pastoral Psychology* 5 (October 1954): 55; Thomas Hennessy and Harold Bluhm, "Using Interest Inventories in Religious and Sacerdotal Counseling," *Catholic Counselor* 2 (1958): 46-49; F. J. Kohler, "Loyola University, National Institute of Mental Health Project on Religion and Mental Health; Report on Research Procedures," *Pastoral Psychology* 10 (February 1959): 44-46; Sr. Estelle, "Psychological Procedures in Guidance," *Catholic School Journal* 54 (October 1954): 255-70; A. A. Zellner, "Screening of Candidates for the Priesthood and Religious Life," *Catholic Educational Review* 58 (February 1960): 96-105.

158.   "Moral Aspects of Tests Used in Guidance," *Catholic Counselor* 2 (Winter 1958): 67-68; A. Dasseau, "An Item Analysis of Responses of Public and Private High School Groups on MMPI," *Catholic Counselor* 3 (1958): 7-9, 29; H. Beir, "Construction of a Rating Scale for the Personality Trait of Willfulness in High School Boys," Abs. *Catholic Educational Review* 45 (October 1958): 483.

159.   Richard P. Vaughn, "Referring Students to Psychiatrists and Psychologists," *Catholic Counselor* 3 (Winter 1959): 30-38.

160.   Nathaniel Paollome, "Adjustment, Adaptation and the Sane Society," *Catholic Counselor* 8 (Fall 1963): 8-12.

161.   J. Maguire, "Mental Health for Religious," *National Catholic Guidance Counselors* 9 (Summer 1965): 5-6; P. C. Hugg, "Sound Personality Growth in Religious Candidates," *Catholic Counselor* 7 (Fall 1962): 9-12; T. N. McCarthy, "Psychological Assessment and Religious Vocation," *Catholic Counselor* 4 (Winter 1960): 44-49; Richard P. Vaughn, "A Psychological Assessment Program for Candidates to the Religious Life," *American Catholic Psychological Association* 1 (February 1963): 65-70; John F. Muldoon, "The Role of the Psychologist as a Consultant to Religious Communities," *Catholic Psychological Record* 3 (1963): 39-50; John Evoy and Van F. Christopher, *Personality Development in Religious Life* (New York: Sheed & Ward, 1963); Mother Claudia, "A Sister Looks at

Psychological Screening of Candidates," *Catholic Counselor* 8 (Winter 1964): 57-59; J. Maguire, "Mental Health Test for Religious," *National Catholic Guidance Counselors Journal* 9 (Summer 1965): 24-56; Frank J. Kohler, "Screening of Applicants for Religious Life," *Journal of Religion and Health* 3 no. 2 (1964): 161-70.

162.   Arlene Marie, "Testing Trio: Testing, Profiles, Counseling," *National Catholic Guidance Counselors Journal* 9 (Winter 1965): 127-9; Sr. Patrick, "Identifying the Emotionally Disturbed," *Catholic School Journal* 65 (October 1965): 47-8.

163.   Alan K. Greenwald, "Reviewing the Psychologist's Report with Seminarians," *Review for Religious* 23 (1964): 602-5.

164.   George Morton, "An Experiment on the Recall of Religious Material," *Religion in Life* 19 (1950): 589-94; Andre Godin and S. Martte, "Magic, Mentality and Sacramental Life in Children of 8 to 14 Years," *Luman Vitae* 60 (1960): 277-96; Mary Amarota, "Needed Research on Religious Development During Adolescence," *Catholic Psychological Record* 2 no. 2 (1963): 1-9; Ralph F. Dunn, "Personality Pattern Among Religious Personnel: A Review," *Catholic Psychological Record* 3 no. 2 (1965): 125-37.

165.   J. B. Maller, "Attitudes of Jewish Students," Pamphlet (New York: Union of American Hebrew Congregations, 1931); M. Nathan, *The Attitude of the Jewish Student in the Colleges and Universities Towards His Religion: A Social Study of Religious Changes* (New York: Block Publishing Co., 1923); M. Kliegsberg, "American-Jewish Soldiers on Jews and Judaism," *YIVO Annual Jewish Social Sciences* 5 (1950): 256-65; L. Lehrer, "Jewish Belongingness of Jewish Youth," *YIVO Annual Jewish Social Sciences* 9 (1954): 137-65; Aaron Savin, "Self-Acceptance of Jewishness by Young Jewish People," *Jewish Education* 26 (December 1955): 22-31; Samuel Glasner, *A Self Survey of a Congregation's Social Attitudes* (New York: Union of American Hebrew Congregations, 1959).

166.   K. S. Pinson, ed., *Essays on Anti-Semitism* (New York: Jewish Social Studies, 1935); T. Graeber and H. Britt, eds., *Jews in a Gentile World* (New York: Macmillan, 1942); Henry Cohen, "Prejudice Reduction in Religious Education," *Religious Education* 59 (1964): 386-89.

Chapter Ten

1.   Walter Kanis, "Healthy Defensiveness in Theological Students," *Ministerial Studies* 1 no. 4 (1967): 3-20; Allen H. Nauss, "The Ministerial Personality: On Avoiding a Stereotype," *Journal of Counseling Psychology* 15 (1968): 1-2.

2.   Robert L. Williams and Cole Spurgion, "Religiosity, Generalized Anxiety and Apprehension Concerning Death," *Journal of Social Psychology* 75 no. 1 (1968): 11-17.

3.   Roger Sheenland, "The Development of a Religious Neuroticism Inventory," *Proceedings of the Christian Association for Psychological Studies* (April 1968): 96-106; Joel Allision, "Adaptive Regression and Intense Religious Experience," *Journal of Nervous and Mental Disease* 145 no. 6 (1967): 452-63.

4. Paul W. Pruyser, "Psychological Examination: Augustine," *Journal for the Scientific Study of Religion* 5 (1965): 284-89.

5. Andrew R. Eickhoff, "A Psychoanalytic Study of St. Paul's Theology of Sex," *Pastoral Psychology* 18 (April 1967): 35-42.

6. Bernard L. Pacella, "A Critical Appraisal of Pastoral Counseling," *American Journal of Psychiatry* 123 no. 6 (1966): 646-51.

7. Gothard Booth, "The Cancer Patient and the Minister," *Pastoral Psychology* 17 (February 1966): 1-5.

8. J. Stanley Glen, *Erich Fromm: A Protestant Critique* (Philadelphia: Westminister Press, 1966).

9. Duane Parker, "Pastoral Consultation Through a Community Mental Health Center," *Pastoral Psychology* 17 (May 1966): 42-47.

10. David R. Mace, "Education and Preparation for Marriage: New Approaches," *Pastoral Psychology* 24 (Fall 1975): 9-16.

11. Joel Allison, "Recent Empirical Studies of Religious Conversion Experiences," *Pastoral Psychology* 17 (September 1966): 21-34.

12. Andre Godin, "Transference in Pastoral Counseling," *Pastoral Psychology* 17 (April 1966): 7-12.

13. Carlo Weber, *The Time of the Fugitive* (Garden City, Long Island: Doubleday & Co., 1971), p. 171.

14. Sharon MacIsaacs, *Freud and Original Sin* (New York: Paulist Press, 1974), p. 107.

15. Ibid.

16. Vincent V. Heir, "Mental Health Training in Catholic Seminaries," *Journal of Religion and Health* 5 no. 1 (1966): 27-34.

17. Le Roy A. Warwick, "The Clergy as Marriage Counselors," *Journal of Religion and Health* 5 no. 3 (1966): 2-9.

18. Jack Bemporad, "Judaism and Psychiatry," in Arieti, pp. 100-108.

19. Erich Fromm, *Psychoanalysis and Religion* (New Haven: Yale University Press, 1950).

20. Philip Reif, *The Triumph of the Therapeutic* (New York: Harper and Row, 1966).

Bibliography

General Books and Monographs

Arieti, Silvano, ed. *American Handbook of Psychiatry*. Vol. 1. New York: Basic Books, 1974.

Barbour, C. E. *Sin and the New Psychology*. New York: Abingdon Press, 1930.

Bemporad, Jack. "Judaism and Psychiatry." In *American Handbook of Psychiatry*. Vol. 1, pp. 100-108. Edited by Silvano Arieti. New York, Basic Books, 1974.

Boisen, Anton T. *The Exploration of the Inner World: A Study of Mental Disorder and Religious Experience*. Chicago: Willett, Clark, 1936.

Boring, Edwin G. *History of Experimental Psychology*. 2nd ed. New York: Appleton-Century-Crofts, Inc., 1950.

Bowers, Margaretta K. *Conflicts of the Clergy*. New York: Thomas Nelson and Sons, 1963.

Brenner, Charles. *An Elementary Textbook of Psychoanalysis*. Garden City, New York: Anchor Books, 1974.

Brill, A. A., ed. *The Basic Writings of Sigmund Freud*. New York: Modern Library, Random House, Inc., 1938.

Brown, James A. C. *Freud and the Post Freudians*. London: Penguin Books, Ltd., 1974.

Burke, Henry R. *Personality Traits of Successful Minor Seminarians*. Washington, D. C.: Catholic University Press, 1947.

Clark, E. T. *The Psychology of Religious Awakening*. New York: MacMillian, 1929.

Cole, William Graham. *Sex and Christianity*. New York: Oxford University Press, 1955.

Cooper, C. *Seven Psychological Portraits: A Handbook for Parents and Teachers*. Milwaukee: Morehouse, 1928.

Darwin, Charles. *On the Origin of Species*. Chicago: Encyclopedia Britannica Press, 1955.

Dicks, Russell C. *Pastoral Work and Personal Counseling*. rev. ed. New York: MacMillan, 1949.

Eissler, Ruth S., et al. *The Psychoanalytic Study of the Child*. Vol. 4. New York: International Universities Press, 1927.

Evoy, John and Christopher, Van F. *Personality Development in Religious Life.* New York: Sheed and Ward, 1963.

Fine, Reuben. *Freud: A Critical Re-Evaluation of his Theories.* New York: David McKay Co. , 1962.

Franzblau, Abraham H. "Psychiatry and Religion." In *Judaism and Psychiatry,* pp. 183-92. Edited by Simon Noveck. New York: Basic Books, 1956.

Freud, Sigmund. *Civilization and Its Discontents.* London: Hogarth Press, 1930.

_____. *Future of an Illusion.* London: Hogarth Press, 1928.

_____. *Moses and Monotheism.* New York: Alfred A. Knopf. 1949.

_____. *The Standard Edition of the Works of Sigmund Freud.* Edited by James Strachey. London: Hogarth Press, 1953-1974.

_____. *Beyond the Pleasure Principle.* In *The Standard Edition of the Works of Sigmund Freud.* Edited by James Strachey. Vol. 18, pp. 3-64. London: Hogarth Press, 1955.

_____. *Group Psychology and Analysis of the Ego.* In *The Standard Edition of the Works of Sigmund Freud.* Edited by James Strachey. Vol. 18, pp. 67-143. London: Hogarth Press, 1955.

_____. *Interpretation of Dreams.* In *The Standard Edition of the Works of Sigmund Freud.* Edited by James Strachey. Vols. 4-5. London: Hogarth Press, 1956.

_____. *Mourning and Melancholia.* In *The Standard Edition of the Works of Sigmund Freud.* Edited by James Strachey. Vol. 14, pp. 239-58. London: Hogarth Press, 1957.

_____. *Psychopathology of Everyday Life.* In *The Standard Edition of the Works of Sigmund Freud.* Edited by James Strachey. Vol. 6. London: Hogarth Press, 1960.

_____. *Studies in Hysteria.* In *The Standard Edition of the Works of Sigmund Freud.* Edited by James Strachey. Vol. 1. London: Hogarth Press, 1953.

_____. *Totem and Taboo.* In *The Standard Edition of the Works of Sigmund Freud.* Edited by James Strachey. Vol. 13, pp. 1-161. London: Hogarth Press, 1957.

Fromm, Erich, *Psychoanalysis and Religion.* New Haven: Yale University Press, 1950.

Gemelli, Agostino. *Psychoanalysis Today.* New York: Kennedy, 1955.

Ginsburg, Sol W. *Man's Place in God's World: A Psychiatric Evaluation.* Cincinnati: Hebrew Union College – Jewish Institute of Religion, 1948.

Glasner, Samuel. *A Self Survey of a Congregation's Social Attitudes.* New York: Union of American Hebrew Congregations, 1959.

Glen, J. Stanley. *Erich Fromm: A Protestant Critique.* Philadelphia: Westminister Press, 1966.

Gold, Henry Raphael. "Can We Speak of Jewish Neuroses?" In *Judaism and Psychiatry,* pp. 155-60. Edited by Simon Noveck. New York: Basic Books, 1956.

Graeber, T. and Britt. M., eds. *Jews in a Gentile World.* New York: Macmillan, 1942.

Hale, Nathan G. *Freud and the Americans: The Beginnings of Psychoanalysis in the United States, 1876-1917.* New York: Oxford University Press, 1971.

Hall, Calvin S., and Lindzey, Gardiner. *Theories of Personality.* New York: John Wiley and Sons. 1957.

Hawthorne, Berkley. *A Critical Analysis of Protestant Church Counseling Centers.* Boston: Boston University, 1960.

Herring, P. B. *Mind Surgery.* Holyoke, Mass.: Elizabeth Thorne Co., 1931.

Hiltner, Seward. *The Christian Shepherd.* New York: Abingdon Press. 1959.

_____. ed. *Constructive Aspects of Anxiety.* New York: Abingdon Press, 1963.

_____. *Pastoral Counseling.* Nashville, Tennessee: Abingdon Cokesbury Press, 1949.

_____. and Colston, Lowell. *The Context of Pastoral Counseling.* New York: Abingdon Press, 1961.

Hulme, William E. *Counseling and Theology.* Philadelphia: Muhlenberg, 1956.

James, William. *Varieties of Religious Experience.* New York: Random House, Inc., 1929.

Jones, Ernest. *The Life and Work of Sigmund Freud.* Edited by L. Trilling and S. Marcus. New York: Basic Books, 1961.

Jorden, A. J. *A Short Psychology of Religion.* New York: Harpers, 1927.

Kagan, Henry Enoch. "Fear and Anxiety: A Jewish View." In *Judaism and Psychiatry,* pp. 45-47. Edited by Simon Noveck. New York: Basic Books, 1956.

Kairys, David. "Conscience and Guilt: A Psychiatric View." In *Judaism and Psychiatry,* pp. 13-23. Edited by Simon Noveck. New York: Basic Books, 1956.

Kinsey, Alfred C. *Sexual Behavior in the Human Female.* Philadelphia: W. B. Saunders Co., 1953.

_____. *Sexual Behavior in the Human Male.* Philadelphia: W. B. Saunders Co., 1948.

Lhota, Brian. *Vocational Interest of Catholic Priests in Studies in Psychology and Psychiatry.* Washington, D. C.: Catholic University Press, 1948.

Liebman, Joshua Loth. *Peace of Mind.* New York: Simon and Schuster, 1946.

Link, H. C. *The Return to Religion.* New York: Macmillan, 1936.

Linn, Louis. "The Need to Believe." In *Judaism and Psychiatry*, pp. 129-34. Edited by Simon Noveck. New York: Basic Books, 1956.

MacIsaacs, Sharon. *Freud and Original Sin.* New York: Paulist Press. 1974.

Malinowski, Bronislaw. *Argonauts of the Western Pacific.* New York: Dutton, 1961.

Mead, Margaret. *Coming of Age in Samoa.* New York: Mentor, 1963.

_____. *Sex and Temperament in Three Primitive Societies.* New York: W. Morrow and Company, 1935.

Mecklin, J. M. *The Passing of the Saint: A Study of a Cultural Type.* Chicago University Press, 1941.

Mowrer, O. Hobart. *The Crisis in Psychiatry and Religion.* Princeton: Van Nostrand, 1961.

Nathan, M. *The Attitude of the Jewish Student in the Colleges and Universities Toward His Religion: A Social Study of Religious Changes.* New York: Block Publishing Co., 1923.

Noveck, Simon. "A Jewish View of Grief." *In Judaism and Psychiatry*, pp. 105-12. Edited by Simon Noveck. New York: Basic Books, 1956.

_____. ed. *Judaism and Psychiatry.* New York: Basic Books, 1956.

Oates, Wayne E. *Anxiety in the Christian Experience.* Philadelphia, Westminister Press, 1955.

_____. *Religious Dimensions of Personality.* New York: Associated Press, 1957.

Odenwald, Robert P. and VanderVeldt, James. *Psychiatry and Catholicism.* 2nd ed. New York: Blackstone Division, McGraw Hill, 1958.

Oliver, J. R. *Pastoral Psychiatry and Mental Health.* New York: Scribner, 1932.

Ostow, Mortimer and Scharfstein, Ben Ami. *The Need to Believe: The Psychology of Religion.* New York: International University Press, 1954.

Outler, Albert. *Psychotherapy and the Christian Message.* New York: Harper and Brothers, 1954.

Pinson, K. S., ed. *Essays on Anti-Semitism.* New York: Jewish Social Studies, 1935.

Proceedings of the Sixth International Congress on Philosophy. New York: Longmans Green, 1926.

Reif, Philip, *The Triumph of the Therapeutic.* New York: Harper and Row, 1966.

Roazan, Paul. *Freud and His Followers.* New York: Alfred A. Knopf. 1975.

Ritley, Hector J. "The Value of Religious Education." In *Judaism and Psychiatry*, pp. 143-53. Edited by Simon Noveck. New York: Basic Books, 1956.

Roberts, David E. *Psychotherapy and a Christian View of Man.* New York: Chas. Scribner's and Sons, 1950.

Salman, D. H. "The Psychology of Religious Experience." *R. M. Bucke Memorial Society for the Study of Religious Experience: Proceedings of the First Annual Conference.* Montreal, Canada: np., 1965.

Sandrow, Edward T. "Conscience and Guilt: A Jewish View." In *Judaism and Psychiatry*, pp. 24-31, Edited by Simon Noveck. New York: Basic Books, 1956.

Saperstein, Milton R. "The Meaning of Personal Religious Experience." In *Judaism and Psychiatry*, pp. 119-24. Edited by Simon Noveck. New York: Basic Books, 1956.

Spiro, Jack D. *A Time to Mourn: The Dynamics of Mourning in Judaism.* Cincinnati: Hebrew Union College-Jewish Institute for Religion, 1961.

Steinbach, Alexander Alan. "Depression: A Jewish View." *In Judaism and Psychiatry,* pp. 72-83. Edited by Simon Noveck. New York: Basic Books, 1956.

_____. "Psychiatry and Religion Meet." In *Judaism and Psychiatry*, pp. 169-71. Edited by Simon Noveck. New York: Basic Books, 1956.

Stolz, K. R. *Pastoral Psychology.* Nashville, Tennessee: Cokesbury Press, 1932.

_____. *The Church and Psychotherapy.* New York: Abingdon Cokesbury Press, 1943.

Weber, Carlo. *The Time of the Fugitive.* Garden City, Long Island: Doubleday and Co., 1971.

Willoughby, R. R. *A Handbook of Social Psychology.* Worcester, Mass.: Clark University Press, 1935.

Winchester, B. S. *The Church and Adult Education.* New York: R. R. Smith, 1930.

Wise, Carroll A. *Psychiatry and the Bible.* New York: Harper and Brothers, 1956.

Yellowless, D. *Psychology's Defense of the Faith.* New York: R. R. Smith, 1930.

Zilboorg, Gregory. *Freud and Religion.* Westminister, Maryland: Westminister, 1958.

_____. *Psychoanalysis and Religion.* New York: Farrar, Straus and Cudahy, 1962.

Pamphlet

Maller, J. B. "Attitudes of Jewish Students," New York: Union of American Hebrew Congregations, 1931.

Articles in Periodical Literature

Abearonla, J. V. "Psychologist Looks at the Problem of Psychology and Ethics." *American Catholic Philosophical Association Proceedings* 31 (1957): 106-14.

Alden, Le Roy. "Distortions of a Sense of Guilt." *Pastoral Psychology* 15 (February 1964): 16-26.

Alexander, Franz. "Psychic Determinism and Responsibility."*Bulletin* of *Guild of Catholic Psychiatrists* 1 (December 1962): 31-35.

Allers, Rudolf. "Impediments of the Human Act." *Ecclesiastical Review* 100 (March 1937): 208-16.

_____. "Holding up the Mirror of Psychoanalysis." *Catholic Charities Review* 23 (March 1939): 70-72.

Allison, Joel. "Adaptive Regression and Intense Religious Experience." *Journal of Nervous and Mental Disease* 145 no. 6 (1967): 452-63.

_____. "Recent Empirical Studies of Religious Conversion Experiences." *Pastoral Psychology* 17 (September 1966): 21-34.

Amarota, Mary. "Needed Research on Religious Development During Adolescence." *Catholic Psychological Record* 2 no. 2 (1963): 1-9.

Anderson, G. C. "Partnership of Theologians and Psychiatrists." *Journal of Religion and Health* 13 (October 1963): 50-69.

_____. "Psychiatry's Influence on Religion." *Pastoral Psychology* 7 (September 1956): 745-54.

Andrew, William R. "Faith and Pastoral Counseling." *Journal of Clinical Pastoral Work* 3 no. 2 (1949): 61-82.

Andrus, J. W. "Traits and Characteristics of Young Children." *Religious Education* 24 (1929): 927-29.

Angers, W. "Guidelines for Counselors for MMPI Interpretation." *Catholic Counselor* 7 (Spring 1963): 120-24.

Arbuckle, Donald S. "Therapy is for All." *Journal of Pastoral Care* 6 (Winter 1952): 34-39.

Backus, E. B. "Religion and Mental Health." *Mental Hygiene Review* 1 (1940): 14-18.

Bain, R. "Religious Attitudes of College Students." *American Journal of Sociology* 32 (1927): 766-70.

Beehan, R. C. "Christian Approach to Psychiatry." *Hospital Progress* 29 (April 1948): 29.

Beir, H. "Construction of a Rating Scale for the Personality Trait of Willfulness in High School Boys." *Catholic Educational Review* 45 (October 1958): 485.

Bergendoff, C. "Mod Imagination and Imago Dei." *Lutheran Quarterly* 10 (May 1958): 99-114.

Bergler, Edmund. "Homosexuality: Disease or Way of Life." *Pastoral Psychology* 8 (June 1957): 49-52.

Biddle, W. Earl. "Integration of Religion and Psychiatry." *Pastoral Psychology* 3 (February 1952): 34-41.

Bier, William C. "Goals in Pastoral Counseling." *Pastoral Psychology* 10 (February 1959): 7-13.

_____. "Psychological Tests in the Screening of Candidates in the Minor Seminary." *National Catholic Education Association Bulletin* 51 (August 1954): 128-35.

_____. "Sigmund Freud and the Faith." *America*, 17 November 1956, pp. 192-96.

Binger, Carl. "Moral Implications of Psychoanalysis." *Pastoral Psychology* 6 (December 1955): 19-26.

Bingham, Thomas J. "Moral Responsibility of the Parishioner or Patient." *Journal of Pastoral Care* 6 no. 1 (1952), pp. 46-55.

_____. "Pastoral Ethical Notes on Problems of Masturbation." *Pastoral Psychology* 11 (June 1960): 19-23.

_____. "The Religious Element in Marriage Counseling." *Pastoral Psychology* 2 (March 1951): 14-18.

Bioren, A. B. "The Theory of Perception in Rogerian Theory." *Catholic Education Review* 60 (January 1962): 62.

Blain, Daniel. "Fostering the Mental Health of Ministers." *Pastoral Psychology* 9 (March 1958): 9-18.

Blelzer, Russell B. "The Minister as a Counselor." *Pastoral Psychology* 8 (March 1957): 28-34.

Bobroff, Alvin S. "Religious Psychodrama." *Group Psychotherapy* 16 (1963): 36-38.

Boisen, Anton T. "The Distinctive Task of the Minister." *Pastoral Psychology* 3 (April 1952): 10-15.

_____. "Economic Distress and Religious Experience: A Study of the Holy Rollers." *Psychiatry* 2 (1939): 185-94.

_____. "The Genesis and Significance of Mystical Identification in Cases of Mental Disorders." *Psychiatry* 15 (1952): 287-96.

_____. "Group Therapy: The Elgin Plan." *Pastoral Psychology* 5 (March 1954): 33-38.

_____. "Ideas of Prophetic Mission." *Journal of Pastoral Care* 12 (Spring 1961): xvi-6.

_____. Letter to "Readers Forum." *Pastoral Psychology* 2 (September 1951): 32-34.

_____. "The Minister as Counselor." *Journal of Pastoral Care* 2 (Spring 1948): 13-22.

_____. "The Period of Beginnings." *Journal of Pastoral Care* 5 (Spring 1951): 13-16.

_____. "The Problem of Sin and Salvation in the Light of Psychology." *Journal of Religion and Health* 22 (July 1942): 288-301.

_____. "Psychiatric Approach to the Study of Religion." *Religious Education* 23 (March 1928): 201-207.

_____. "The Service of Worship in a Mental Hospital: Its Therapeutic Significance." *Journal of Clinical Pastoral Work* 2 no. 1 (1948): 19-25.

_____. "The Therapeutic Significance of Anxiety." *Journal of Pastoral Care* 4 (Summer 1951): 1-15.

Bond, Earl D. "Anxiety from the Psychiatrist's Viewpoint." *Pastoral Psychology* 2 (March 1951): 14-21.

Bonnell, John Sutherland. "Anxiety: The Sickness of Western Civilization." *Pastoral Psychology* 8 (May 1957): 1-14.

_____. "Counseling Divorced Persons." *Pastoral Psychology* 9 (June 1958): 11-15.

_____. "Healing for Mind and Body." *Pastoral Psychology* 1 (March 1950): 30-33.

_____. "The Practice of Counseling in the Local Church." *Pastoral Psychology* 11 (February 1960): 24-30.

_____. "Religious Disciplines" *Pastoral Psychology* 1 (February 1950): 17-18.

Booth, Gothard. "Basic Concepts of Psychosomatic Medicine." *Pastoral Psychology* 2 (October 1951): 11-18.

_____. "The Cancer Patient and the Minister." *Pastoral Psychology* 17 (February 1966): 1-5.

_____. "Masturbation." *Pastoral Psychology* 5 (Novenber 1943): 13-20.

_____. "Unconscious Motivation in the Choice of the Ministry." *Pastoral Psychology* 9 (August 1958): 18-24.

Bose, R. G. "Religious Concepts of Children." *Religious Education* 24 (1929): 24.

Boyd, William. "Psychiatrists." *Commonweal*, 7 January 1949, p. 326.

Braceland, Francis. J. "A Psychiatrist Examines the Relationship Between Psychiatry and the Catholic Clergy." *Pastoral Psychology* 10 (February 1959): 14-25.

Brevis, Harry J. "Counseling Prison Inmates." *Pastoral Psychology* 7 (February 1956): 35-42.

Brooks. Charles F. "Some Limiting Factors in Pastoral Counseling." *Pastoral Psychology* 2 (March 1951): 26-31.

Bruder, Ernest E. "Clinical Pastoral Training as a Hospital Medium in Public Relations." *Pastoral Psychology* 4 (November 1953): 27-36.

_____. "A Clinically Trained Religious Ministry in the Mental Hospital." *Quarterly Review of Psychiatry and Neurology* 2 (1947): 543-52.

_____. "Psychotherapy and some of its Theological Implications." *Journal of Pastoral Care* 6 (Summer 1952): 28.

_____. "Some Reflections on Psychiatry and Religion." *Journal of Pastoral Care* 5 (Summer 1951): 30-36.

_____. and Barb, Marion L. "A Survey of 10 Years of Clinical Pastoral Training at St. Elizabeth's Hospital." *Journal of Pastoral Care* 10 (Summer 1956): 86-94.

Burkhart, Roy A. "The Church Program of Education in Marriage and the Family: From Birth to Twelve." *Pastoral Psychology* 2 (November 1951): 10-14.

_____. "Is the Church Authoritarian?" *Pastoral Psychology* 5 (April 1954): 25-28.

_____. "Minister's Own Freedom." *Pastoral Psychology* 1 (March 1950): 10-12.

_____. "A Program of Pre-Marital Counseling." *Pastoral Psychology* 1 (September 1950): 25-34.

Burns, James H. "The Application of Psychology to Preachings." *Pastoral Psychology* 3 (March 1952): 29-33.

_____. "The Institute for Pastoral Care." *Pastoral Psychology* 4 (October 1953): 21-24.

Butler, Donald J. "Theology and Psychology: Some Points of Convergence." *Encounter*, 1958, pp. 31-36.

Cambell, Cajetan. "An Evaluation of Catholic Chaplains' Training." *Guild of Catholic Psychiatrists Bulletin* 6 no. 2 (April 1959): 19-21.

Cannon, T. J. "Function of Psychology Courses in a Catholic College." *Catholic Educational Review* 51 (November 1953): 596-603.

Carelton, N. "Pre-Registration Guidance in Catholic Colleges." *Catholic Educational Review* 40 (1942): 162-68.

Carrier, Blanche. "Counseling Pre-Ministerial Students." *Pastoral Psychology* 2 (November 1951): 21-25.

Cesarman, F. C. "The Conversion of Sex Offenders During Psychotherapy: Two Cases." *Journal of Pastoral Care* 11 (Spring 1957): 25-35.

Chamberlin, J. Maxwell. "Readers Forum." *Pastoral Psychology* 7 (April 1956): 54.

Charters, J. A. "The Opportunity of the Church for Sex Education." *Religious Education* 27 (1932): 428-34.

Christensen, Carl W. "Religious Conversion In Adolescence." *Pastoral Psychology* 16 (September 1965): 17-36.

_____. "Role of the Psychiatrist Consultant to a Seminary." *Journal of Pastoral Care* 9 (Spring 1955): 1-7.

The Church and Mental Retardation. Pastoral Psychology 13 (September 1962).

Clark, A. W. "Toad's Eye View of Psychiatry and Faith." *Journal of Religion and Health* 2 (July 1963), 296-312.

Clark, Walter Houston. "The Psychology of Religion and the Understanding of Man in Religious Education." *Religious Education* 54 (1959): 18-23.

Claudia, Mother. "A Sister Looks at Psychological Screening of Candidates." *Catholic Counselor* 8 (Winter 1964): 57-59.

Clinebell, Howard J. "American Protestantism and the Problem of Alcoholism." *Journal of Clinical Pastoral Work* 3 no. 1 (1949): 199-215.

_____. "The Challenge of the Speciality of Pastoral Counseling." *Pastoral Psychology* 15 (April 1964): 17-28.

_____. "Ego Psychology and Pastoral Counseling." *Pastoral Psychology* 14 (February 1963): 26-36.

_____. "Pastoral Care of the Alcoholic's Family Before Sobriety." *Pastoral Psychology* 13 (April 1962): 19-29.

Coe, George A. "What Constitutes a Scientific Interpretation of Religion?" *Journal of Religion* 6 (May 1926): 225-35.

Cohen, Henry. "Prejudice Reduction in Religious Education." *Religious Education* 59 (1964): 386-89.

Commins, W. P. "What May We Expect of Gestalt Psychology?" *Catholic Educational Review* 35 (March 1937): 135-43.

"Consultation Clinic." *Pastoral Psychology* 2 (September 1951): 41-51.

"Consultation Clinic." *Pastoral Psychology* 5 (April 1954): 57-58.

"Consultation Clinic: How Far Can A Pastor Go With an Extreme Neurotic?" *Pastoral Psychology* 2 (January 1952): 49-55.

"Consultation Clinic: Masturbation." *Pastoral Psychology* 11 (May 1960): 51-71.

"Consultation Clinic: The Pastor and Suicide." *Pastoral Psychology* 4 (December 1953): 51-54.

Cooley, Ewing C. and Hutton, Jerry B. "Adolescent Religious Response to Religious Appeal as Related to IPAT Anxiety." *Journal of Social Psychology* 67 no. 2 (1965): 325-27.

"Cooperation Between Priests and Alienists," *Catholic Charities Review* 33 (January 1939): 14-15.

Currian, Charles A. "A Catholic Psychologist Looks at Pastoral Counseling." *Pastoral Psychology* 10 (February 1959): 21-28.

_____. "The Counseling Relationship." *Journal of Counseling Psychology* 6 (1959): 266-70.

_____. "Religious Factors and Values in Counseling." *Catholic Counselor* 3 (1958): 3-5, 24.

D'Agnostino, C. "Mental Hygiene and the Clergy." *Catholic Charities Review* 33 (May 1949): 116-19.

Daim, Wilfred. "On Depth-Psychology and Salvation." *Journal of Psychiatry and Religion*, Proceedings 2 (1952): 24-37.

Dasseau, A. "An Item Analysis of Responses of Public and Private High School Groups on MMPI." *Catholic Counselor* 3 (1958): 7-9, 29.

Davies, K. "What Everyone Should Know About Psychiatry." *Catholic Charities Review* 34 (May 1950): 114-16.

de Hass, C. H. "Psychology and Religion." *Cross Currents* 4 (Fall 1953): 70-75.

Deitchman, Robert. "The Evolution of a Ministerial Counseling Center." *Journal of Pastoral Care* 11 (Winter 1957): 7-14.

De Nardo, R. A. "Depth Psychology and the Contribution of Existential Synthesis." *New Scholastic* 32 (April 1958): 187-201.

Dicks, Russell C. "The Hospital Chaplain." *Pastoral Psychology* 1 (March 1950): 50-54.

_____. "Sacrament of Conversation." *Pastoral Psychology* 2 (May 1951): 17-21.

Dodd, Aleck. "Relationship Therapy as Religion." *Journal of Psychotherapy and Religion*, *Proceedings* 1 (1954): 41-51.

Dodds, Robert C. "A Parochial Evaluation of Clinical Pastoral Training." *Journal of Pastoral Care* 2 (Fall 1948): 22-25.

Dohen, D. "Unless a Man Be Born Again." *Integrity* 6 (October 1951): 34-40.

Dolard, John and Miller, Neale E. "Free Association Without Understanding the Past." *Pastoral Psychology* 3 (February 1952): 31-34.

Dougherty, E. O. "Religion and Psychology." *Catholic Mind* 49 (November 1951): 739-44.

Doyle, Robert E. "Guidance Services in Metropolitan Catholic Schools: A Status Report." *National Catholic Guidance Conference Journal* 9 (1965): 227-29.

Dunbar, H. F. "Mental Hygiene and Religious Teaching." *Mental Hygiene* 19 (1935): 535-37.

Dunn, Ralph F. "Personality Pattern Among Religious Personnel: A Review." *Catholic Psychological Record* 3 no. 2 (1965): 125-37.

Duvall, Sylvanus M. "Sex Morals in the Context of Religion." *Pastoral Psychology* 3 (May 1952): 33-37.

Eastman, Fred. "Father of the Clinical Pastoral Movement." *Journal of Pastoral Care* 7 (Spring 1953): 3-7.

Editorial. *Journal of Pastoral Care* 1 (Winter 1947): 33.

Editorial. *Pastoral Psychology* 1 (May 1950): 9-15.

Eickhoff, Andrew R. "A Psychoanalytic Study of St. Paul's Theology of Sex." *Pastoral Psychology* 18 (April 1967): 35-42.

Estelle, Sr. "Psychological Procedures in Guidance." *Catholic School Journal* 154 (October 1954): 255-70.

Evenson, George O. "Reader's Forum." *Pastoral Psychology* 4 (May 1953): 54.

Fahs, S. C. "How Childish Should a Child's Religion Be." *Religious Education* 24 (1929): 910-17.

Fairbanks, Rollin J. "Cooperation Between Clergy and Psychiatrists." *Journal of Pastoral Care* 1 (Spring-Summer 1947): 5-11.

_____. "Cooperation Between Clergy and Psychiatrists." *Pastoral Psychology* 2 (September 1951): 19-23.

Feldman, Sandor S. "Notes on Some Religious Rites and Ceremonies." *Journal of Hillside Hospital* (1959): 887-92.

Finch, Stuart McIntire. "The Pastor's Role with the Anxious Child." *Pastoral Psychology* 2 (October 1951): 23-28.

_____. and Kroor, Edwin, H., "Some Educational Factors in the Religious Education of Children." *Religious Education* 54 (1959): 36-43.

Fisher, Alden L. "Freud and the Image of Man." *American Catholic Philosophical Association Proceedings* 35 (1961): 45-77.

Fishman, Joshua A. "How Safe is Psychoanalysis?" *Jewish Education* 23 no. 1 (1952): 45-48.

Fletcher, Joseph. "A Moral Philosophy of Sex." *Pastoral Psychology* 4 (February 1953): 31-37.

Ford, John C. "May Catholics be Psychoanalyzed?" *Pastoral Psychology* 5 (October 1954): 25-34.

Forest, I. de. "Restoration of Personal Integrity: The Keynote of Psychoanalytic Therapy." *Journal of Pastoral Care* 6 no. 3 (1952): 45-52.

Foster, Lloyd E. "Religion and Psychiatry." *Pastoral Psychology* 1 (February 1950): 7-13.

Fowler, John Richard. "What the Pastor Should Know About Psychological Tests." *Pastoral Psychology* 15 (March 1964): 24-29.

Frank, Lawrence. Review of *Life Against Death* by Norman O. Brown. *Pastoral Psychology* 10 (December 1959): 74.

Franklin, P. "Measurement of the Comprehensive Difficulty of the Precepts and Parables of Jesus." *University of Iowa Studies: Studies in Character* 2 no. 1 (1967): 63.

Franzblau, Abraham N. "The Ministry of Counseling." *Journal of Pastoral Care* 9 (Autumn 1955): 137-44.

Fromm, Erich. "Freud and Jung." *Pastoral Psychology* 1 (July 1950): 11-15.

_____. "The Philosophy Basic to Freud's Psychoanalysis." *Pastoral Psychology* 13 (February 1962): 26-32.

"Full Time Psychologist: An Experiment." *Catholic School Journal* 39 (February 1939): 41-43.

Furgeson, Earl H. "The Definition of Religious Conversion." *Pastoral Psychology* 16 (September 1965): 8-16.

_____. "Preaching and Counseling Functions of the Minister." *Journal of Pastoral Care* 2 (Winter 1948): 11-18.

_____. "Preaching and Personality." *Pastoral Psychology* 10 (October 1959): 9-14.

Gelberman, J. H. and Koback, D. "Psychology and Modern Hasidism." *Journal of Pastoral Care* 17 (September 1963): 27-30.

George, G. F. "Pope on Psychoanalysis." *America*, 4 October 1952, p. 12.

Gerry, W. J. "Freud Has Passed and Freudianism Also Goes." *America*, October 1939. pp. 616-17.

Girende, Peter P. and Paollome, Nathaniel J. "Client Rapport and the Counselor's Religious Status: an Exploration." *Journal of the National Conference of Catholic Guidance Counselors* 9 no. 4 (1965): 208-19.

Gluckman, Robert M. "The Chaplain as a Member of the Diagnostic Clinical Team." *Journal of Pastoral Care* 8 (Spring 1954): 83-87.

Godin, Andre. "Transference in Pastoral Counseling." *Pastoral Psychology* 17 (April 1966): 7-12.

_____. and Martte, S. "Magic, Mentality and Sacramental Life in Children 8 to 14 Years." *Lumen Vitae* 60 (1960): 277-96.

Golden, Charles P. "Religion and Current Trends in Psychology." *Religious Education* 45 (1950): 331-35.

Golnar, Joseph H. "Dilemma of the American Jew." *Jewish Social Service Quarterly* 31 (1954): 165-73.

Gordon, Stanley. "Personality and Attitude Correlates of Religious Conversion." *Journal for the Scientific Study of Religion* 4 no. 10 (1964): 60-63.

Graebner, Oliver E. "Children's Concepts of God." *Inter-Institutional Seminar in Child Development, Collected Papers* (1957): 184-92.

Graham, A. "Psychological Problems of Maturity." *Pastoral Psychology* 5 (April 1954): 47-54.

Grant, P. McW. "The Moral and Religious Life of the Individual in the Light of the New Psychology." *Mental Hygiene* 12 (1928): 449-91.

Greely, Andrew M. "A Note on the Origins of Religious Differences." *Journal for the Scientific Study of Religion* 3 (1963): 321-31.

Greenwald, Alan K. "Reviewing the Psychologist's Report with Seminarians." *Review for Religious* 23 (1964): 602-605.

Gross, Alfred A. "The Homosexual in Society." *Pastoral Psychology* 1 (March 1950): 38-48.

"Guilt Feelings and Neuroses," *America,* 23 December 1950. p. 350.

Haas, Alfred B. "The Therapeutic Value of Hymns." *Pastoral Psychology* 1 (December 1950): 39-42.

Hall, Calvin S. "Freud's Concept of Anxiety." *Pastoral Psychology* 6 (March 1955): 43-48.

_____. "The Function of the Psychiatric Chaplain." *Journal of Pastoral Care* 9 (August 1955): 145-52.

Harden, W. Review of *Crisis in Psychiatry* by O. Hobart Mowrer. *Christian Century,* 13 September 1961 pp. 1556-58.

Harms, C. "The Nervous Jew: A Study in Social Psychiatry." *Disorders of the Nervous System* 3 (1942): 47-52.

Harrison, Walter R. "A Study of Church Attitudes in the East Baton Rouge Area." *Religious Education* 47 (1952): 39-52.

Hartshorne, H., May, M. et. al. "Testing the Knowledge of Right and Wrong." *Religious Education Monograph* 9 no. 1 (1927): 72.

Hayden, E. C. "Spiritual (Religious) Values and Mental Hygiene." *Mental Hygiene* 14 (1930): 779-90.

Heir, Vincent V. "Mental Health Training in Catholic Seminaries." *Journal of Religion and Health* 5 no. 1 (1966): 27-34.

Hendin, Hubert, "What a Pastor Ought to Know about Suicide." *Pastoral Psychology* 4 (December 1953): 4-5.

Hennessy, Thomas and Bluhm, Harold. "Using Interest Inventories in Religious and Sacerdotal Counseling." *Catholic Counselor* 2 (1958): 46-49.

Higgins, John W. "Some Considerations of Psychoanalytic Theory." *American Catholic Philosophical Association Proceedings* 35 (1961): 21-44.

Higgins, Ralph. "Client-Centered Psychotherapy and Christian Doctrine." *Journal of Pastoral Care* 3 (Spring 1949): 1-12.

"High School Curriculum Should Include Psychology." *Catholic Educational Review* 51 (January 1953): 52.

Hill, William S. "The Psychology of Conversion." *Pastoral Psychology* 6 (November 1955): 43-63.

Hiltner, Seward. "The American Association of Pastoral Counselors: A Critique." *Pastoral Psychology* 15 (April 1964): 8-16.

_____. "The Contributions of Religion to Mental Health." *Mental Hygiene* 24 (1940): 366-77.

_____. "Freud, Psychoanalysis and Religion." *Pastoral Psychology* 7 (November 1956): 9-21.

_____. "Pastoral Psychology and Christian Ethics." *Pastoral Psychology* 4 (April 1953): 23-33.

_____. "Pastoral Psychology and Constructive Theology." *Pastoral Psychology* 4 (June 1953): 17-26.

_____. "Pastoral Psychology and Pastoral Counseling." *Pastoral Psychology* 3 (November 1952): 21-28.

_____. "Reader's Forum." *Pastoral Psychology* 7 (April 1956): 55.

_____. "Religion and Psychoanalysis." *Journal of Pastoral Care* 3 (Spring-Summer 1950): 32-42.

_____. Review of *Practical and Theoretical Aspects of Psychoanalysis* by Lawrence S. Kubic. *Pastoral Psychology* 1 (April 1950): 63-64.

_____. Review of *Psychology of Sex Relations* by Theodor Reik. *Pastoral Psychology* 3 (September 1952): 78-80.

_____. Review of *Religion and the Cure of Souls in Jung's Psychology* by Hans Schaer, translated by R. F. C. Hull. *Pastoral Psychology* 1 (September 1950): 60-61.

Hoffman, J. "Psychological, Pathological Guilt Feelings and Psychiatry." *Journal of Pastoral Care* 6 no. 2 (1952): 42-52.

Hold, Herbert, and Wenich, Charles. "Group Pastoral Counseling." *Pastoral Psychology* 14 (November 1963): 13-22.

Hollander, I. Fred. "The Specific Nature of the Clergy's Role in Mental Health." *Pastoral Psychology* 10 (November 1959): 11-22.

Holt, J. B. "Holiness Religion: Cultural Shock and Social Reorganization." *American Sociological Review* 5 (1940): 740-47.

Horney, Karen. "The Search for Glory." *Pastoral Psychology* 1 (September 1950): 13-20.

Howard, Judson D. "Churches and Mental Illness." *Pastoral Psychology* 4 (October 1953): 35-38.

Howe, Revel L. "The Crucial and Correlative Role of Pastoral Theology." *Pastoral Psychology* 11 (February 1960): 37-44.

Huber, Milton J. "Counseling the Single Woman." *Pastoral Psychology* 10 (April 1959): 11-18.

Hugg. P. C. "Sound Personality Growth in Religious Candidates." *Catholic Counselor* 7 (Fall 1962): 9-12.

Hyde, C. W. and Leslie, Robert C. "Introduction to Group Therapy for Graduate Students ." *Journal of Pastoral Care* 6 no. 2 (1952): 19-27.

Jackson, Joan K. "Alcoholism as a Family Crisis." *Pastoral Psychology* 13 (April 1962): 8-18.

Jeanette, M., Sister, "Psychoanalysis." *Catholic School Journal* 31 (April 1931): 130-32.

Johnson, Paul E. "Christian Love and Self Love." *Pastoral Psychology* 2 (March 1951): 14-20.

_____. "Contributions of Psychology to the Teacher of Religion." *Journal of Bible and Religion* 24 (July 1956): 167-72.

_____. "Jesus as a Practicing Psychologist." *Pastoral Psychology* 2 (December 1951): 17-21.

_____. "The Lonely Person." *Pastoral Psychology* 8 (June 1957): 41-48.

_____. "Methods of Pastoral Counseling." *Journal of Pastoral Care* 1 no. 1 (1947): 27-32.

_____. "Religious Psychology and Health." *Mental Hygiene* 31 (1947): 556-66.

Jung, Carl. "Psychotherapist of the Clergy." *Pastoral Psychology* 7 (April 1956): 25-42.

Kagan, Enoch. "The Rabbi and the Community." *Journal of Religion and Health* 13 (July 1950): 50-61.

_____. "The Role of the Rabbi as Counselor." *Pastoral Psychology* 5 (October 1954): 17-23.

Kanis, Walter. "Healthy Defensiveness in Theological Students." *Ministerial Studies* 1 no. 4 (1967): 3-20.

Kant, M. "Of Cabbages and Cats." *Catholic World* 156 (January 1943): 438-47.

Katz, Robert L. "Aspects of Pastoral Psychology and the Rabbinate." *Pastoral Psychology* 5 (October 1954): 35-42.

Keenan, A. "What Can be Done to a Neurosis." *Integrity* 5 (May 1951): 26-32.

Kelly, W. A. "Preparation of the Instructor in Educational Psychology." *Catholic Educational Review* 52 (February 1954): 102-12.

Kennedy, W. J. "Psychiatric Tests for Seminarians." *National Catholic Education Association Bulletin* 51 (August 1954): 89-95.

Kew, Clifton E. "Group Healing in the Church." *Pastoral Psychology* 5 (March 1954): 44-50.

_____. "Group Psychotherapy in a Church Setting." *Pastoral Psychology* 1 (January 1951): 31-37.

_____. and Kew, Clinton J. "Principles and Values of Group Psychotherapy Under Church Auspices." *Pastoral Psychology* 6 (April 1955): 37-48.

Kildahl, P. "The Personalities of Sudden Religious Converts." *Pastoral Psychology* 16 (September 1965): 37-44.

Kirkendull, Lester. "Premarital Sex Relations: The Problem and Its Implications." *Pastoral Psychology* 7 (April 1956): 45-56.

Kirkpatrick, M. E. "Mental Hygiene and Religion." *Mental Hygiene* 24 (1940): 378-89.

Kliegsberg, M. "American-Jewish Soldiers on Jews and Judaism." *YIVO Annual Jewish Social Sciences* 5 (1950): 256-65.

Kling, Frederick. "A Study of Testing as Related to the Ministery." *Religious Education* 53 (1958): 243-48.

_____. "Value Structures and the Minister's Purpose." *Pastoral Psychology* 12 (March 1961): 13-23.

Knight, James A. "Calvinism and Psychoanalysis: A Comparative Study." *Pastoral Psychology* 13 (December 1963): 10-17.

_____. "The Use and Misuses of Religion by the Emotionally Disturbed." *Pastoral Psychology* 13 (March 1962): 8-10.

Koberle, Adolph. "The Problem of Guilt." translated by John W. Duberstein. *Pastoral Psychology* 8 (December 1957): 33-39.

Kohler, Frank J. "Loyola University National Institute of Mental Health Project on Religion and Mental Health: Report on Research Procedures." *Pastoral Psychology* 10 (February 1959): 44-46.

_____. "Screening of Applicants for Religious Life." *Journal of Religion and Health* 3 no. 2 (1964): 161-70.

Krill, Donald F. "Psychoanalysts, Mowrer and the Existentialists." *Pastoral Psychology* 6 (October 1965): 27-36.

Kubie, Lawrence S. "Psychoanalysis and Healing Faith." *Pastoral Psychology* 1 (March 1950): 13-18.

Kuether, Frederick C. "The Council for Clinical Training." *Pastoral Psychology* 4 (October 1953): 17-20.

Kurich, Joseph. "Psychiatric and Psychological Selection of Candidates for the Sisterhood." *Guild of Catholic Psychiatrists Bulletin* 1 (1960): 19-25.

Landis, Carney P. "Psychotherapy and Religion." *Review of Religion* 10 (1946): 413-24.

_____. "Psychotherapy and Religion." *Journal of Pastoral Care* 1 (Spring-Summer 1947): 19-27.

Landon, P. "Psychotherapists and the New Clergy." *Christian Century*, 26 April 1961, pp. 515-16.

Lehrer, L. "Jewish Belongingness of Jewish Youth." *YIVO Annual Jewish Social Sciences* 9 (1954): 137-65.

Leonard, E. A. "Counseling in the Catholic High Schools of the Middle Western States." *Catholic Educational Review* 44 (1946): 483-91.

Leslie, Robert C. "Group Therapy: A New Approach for the Church." *Journal of Pastoral Care* 5 (Spring 1951): 36-45.

_____. "Pastoral Group Therapy." *Journal of Pastoral Care* 6 no. 2 (1952): 56-61.

Lester, Kim Edward. "A Critical Study of Selective Changes in Protestant Theological Students with Clinical Pastoral Education: Report on Doctoral Dissertations." *Pastoral Psychology* 13 (March 1962): 39-40.

Levine, Milton I. and Howe, Reuel L. "Pediatrics and the Church: A Symposium." *Journal of Pastoral Care* 3 (Fall-Winter 1949) 39-44.

Levinson, Boris M. "The Intelligence of Applicants for Admission to Jewish Day Schools." *Jewish Social Studies* 19 (1957): 129-40.

Levy, Ruth. "The Implications of Psychiatry for Religion." *Reconstructionist* 16 (1951): 26-29.

Lewin, Herbert S. "The Use of Religious Elements in Modern Psychotherapy." *Journal of Pastoral Care* 3 (Fall-Winter 1950): 9-16.

Leys, W. A. R. "Soul Saving in the Light of Modern Psychology." *Religious Education* 25 (1930): 344-49.

Ligon, Ernest M. "Possible Contributions of Recent Researchers in Psychology to Religious Education." *Religious Education* 44 (1949): 211-16.

_____. "A Plea for the Child," *Presbyterian Tribune* 23 (January 1934): 51.

Limaco, F. M. "Religious Values Must be Acknowledged by Today's Psychologists." *Catholic School Journal* 60 (April 1960): 38-39.

Lindeman, Erich. "Symptomology and Management of Acute Grief." *Pastoral Psychology* 14 (September 1963): 8-18.

Linn, Louis and Schwarz, Leo M. "The Domains of Psychiatry and Religion." *Pastoral Psychology* 9 (October 1958): 41-49.

Londin, Perry, et al. "Religion, Guilt and Ethical Standards." *Journal of Social Psychology* 63 (December 1964): 145-59.

Loomis, Earl. "Child Psychiatry and Religion." *Pastoral Psychology* 7 (September 1956): 27-33.

Loper, Vere V. "A Christian Tries to Hold Homes Together." *Pastoral Psychology* 8 (December 1957): 9-14.

Luschermer, Paul. "Responsibility and Its Relation to Personality Problems." *Pastoral Psychology* 1 (May 1950): 16-22.

McAllister, J. B. "Psychoanalysis and Morality." *New Scholastic* 30 (July 1956): 10-29.

McCarthy, T. N. "Psychological Assessment and Religious Vocation." *Catholic Counselor* 4 (Winter 1960): 44-49.

McClelland, D. C. "Religious Overtones in Psychoanalysis." *Theology Today* 16 (April 1959): 40-64.

McCormick, C. G. "The Emotions and a Positive Morality." *Religious Education* 42 (1947): 271-74.

McDonough, A. "Reliable Psychotherapy." *Sign* 28 (July 1949): 33.

Mace, David R. "Education and Preparation for Marriage: New Approaches." *Pastoral Psychology* 24 (Fall 1975): 9-16.

_____. "The Minister's Role in Marriage Preparation." *Pastoral Psychology* 3 (May 1952): 45-48.

McNamee, Finlan. "Religion and Psychiatry." *Hospital Progress* 40 (September 1960): 62-65.

McNeill, Harry. "Freudians and Catholics." *Commonweal* 46 (1946): 350-53.

Madden, Myron C. "The Crisis of Becoming a Christian." *Pastoral Psychology* 2 (May 1951): 28-31.

Maguire, J. "Mental Health for Religious." *National Catholic Guidance Counselors Bulletin* 9 (Summer 1965): 5-6.

_____. "Mental Health Test for Religious." *National Catholic Guidance Counselors Journal* 9 (Summer 1965): 24-56.

Mahoney, Vincent. "Scrupulosity from the Psychoanalytic Viewpoint." *Guild of Catholic Psychiatrists Bulletin* 2 (December 1957) 11-21.

Malzberg, B. "New Data Relative to the Incidence of Mental Disease Among Jews." *Mental Hygiene* 20 (1936): 80-91.

Marie, Arlene. "Testing Trio: Testing, Profiles, Counseling," *National Catholic Guidance Counselors Journal* 9 (Winter 1965): 127-29.

Maritain, Jacques. "Freudianism and Psychoanalysis." *Cross Currents* 6 (Fall 1956): 307-24.

Marriott, V. E. "New Flowers of the Spirit." *Religious Education* 24 (1929): 250-62.

Martin, J. M. "Opportunities for the Catholic Psychiatrist." *American Ecclesiastical Review* 135 (August 1956): 37-86.

Masserman, Jules H. and Palmer, Ralph T. "Psychiatric and Psychological Tests for Ministerial Personnel." *Pastoral Psychology* 12 (March 1961): 24-31.

May, Rollo. "The Healing Power of Symbols." *Pastoral Psychology* 11 (November 1960): 37-49.

_____. "Religion and Anxiety." *Pastoral Psychology* 1 (March 1950): 46-49.

_____. "Religion, Psychotherapy, and the Achievement of Selfhood." *Pastoral Psychology* 2 (October 1951): 26-33.

_____. "Religion, Psychotherapy, and the Achievement of Selfhood." *Pastoral Psychology* 2 (November 1951): 15-20.

_____. "Religion, Psychotherapy, and the Achievement of Selfhood." *Pastoral Psychology* 2 (January 1952): 26-33.

_____. "Religion: Source of Strength or Weakness?" *Pastoral Psychology* 4 (February 1953): 68-73.

_____. "Toward an Understanding of Anxiety." *Pastoral Psychology* 1 (March 1950): 25-31.

Melamed, I. M. "The Jewish Prisoner." *Jewish Social Service Quarterly* 31 (1954): 173-79.

Menninger, Karl. "The Character of the Therapist." *Pastoral Psychology* 9 (November 1958): 14-18.

_____. "Kinsey's Study of Sexual Behavior in the Human Male and Female." *Pastoral Psychology* 5 (February 1954) 43-85.

_____. "Religion and Psychiatry." *Pastoral Psychology* 2 (September 1951): 10-18.

_____. "Reply." *Commonweal*, 30 May 1952, pp. 200-201.

Menninger, William C. "Psychiatry and Religion." *Pastoral Psychology* 1 (February 1950): 14-16.

Meyer, Adolf. "Repression, Freedom and Discipline." *Pastoral Psychology* 7 (September 1956): 13-18.

Meyers, A. J. "Use of Fear in Religious Education." *Religious Education* 18 (1923): 908-13.

Miller, Charles. "The Significance of the Center of Community Organization in Metropolitan Communities." *Jewish Social Service Quarterly* 27 (1950): 53-61.

Miller, Randolf Crump. "Anxiety and Learning." *Pastoral Psychology* 15 (February 1964): 66-75.

Miller, Samuel H. "Exploring the Boundary Between Religion and Psychiatry." *Journal of Pastoral Care* 6 (Summer 1952): 1-11.

"Ministering to the Mind," *America*, 2 August 1947, pp. 482-83.

Mode, Doris. "God-Centered Therapy: A Criticism of Client-Centered Therapy." *Journal of Pastoral Care* 4 (Spring-Summer (1950): 19-23.

Moller, Herbert. "Affective Mysticism in Western Civilization." *Psychoanalytic Review* 52 (1965): 115-30.

Molligen, A. T. "Utilization of Religious Attitudes in Clinical Psychiatry." *Bulletin of the Isaac Ray Medical Library* 2 (1954): 116-35.

Montagu, Ashley. "The Origins of Love and Hate." *Pastoral Psychology* 4 (December 1953): 46-48.

"Moral Aspects of Tests Used in Guidance." *Catholic Counselor* 2 (Winter 1958): 67-68.

Morgan, Norman C. "Religion in Psychotherapy." *Pastoral Psychology* 8 (October 1957): 17-22.

Morris, C. W. "The Terror of Good Works." *Pastoral Psychology* 8 (July 1957): 25-32.

Morton, George. "An Experiment on the Recall of Religious Material." *Religion in Life* 19 (1950): 589-94.

Mowrer, O. Hobart. Review of *Crisis in Psychiatry* by W. Harden. *Christian Century*, 13 September 1961, p. 1080.

_____. "Transference and Scrupulosity." *Journal of Religion and Health* 23 (July 1963): 3-43.

Moynihan, James F. "Student Counseling in Catholic Education." *Higher Education* 18 (1947): 154-58.

Muldoon, John F. "The Role of the Psychologist as a Consultant to Religious Communities." *Catholic Psychological Record* 3 (1965): 39-50.

Murphy, Carrol. "The Ministry of Counseling." *Pastoral Psychology* 8 (December 1957): 15-32.

Murray, John B. "Personality Study of Priests and Seminarians." *Homiletic and Pastoral Review* 49 (1958): 443-47.

Nauss, Allen H. "The Ministerial Personality: On Avoiding a Stereotype." *Journal of Counseling Psychology* 15 (1968): 1-2.

Nichols, Roger B. "Anxiety: An Investigation in Diagnosis and Christian Therapy." *Journal of Pastoral Care* 2 (Winter 1948): 19-26.

Niebuhr, Reinhold. "The Christian Moral Witness and Some Disciplines of Modern Culture." *Pastoral Psychology* 11 (February 1960): 45-54.

Nording, R. B. "Man's Rationality: A Psychological View." *Catholic Educational Review* 55 (February 1957): 73-81.

"Notes and News." *Pastoral Psychology* 5 (October 1954): 55.

Novis, K. "Cure All: Psychoanalysis." *Catholic World* 167 (June 1948): 218-22.

Oates, Wayne E. "The Helping and Hindering Power of Religion." *Pastoral Psychology* 6 (May 1955): 41-49.

_____. "Levels of Pastoral Care: The New Testament Concept of a Health-Giving Ministry." *Pastoral Psychology* 2 (May 1951): 11-16.

_____. "Pastoral Psychology in the South" *Pastoral Psychology* 2 (May 1961): 9-10.

_____. Review of *Christianity and Fear: A Study in History* and *The Psychology and Hygiene of Religion*, by Oskar Pfister, Translated by W. H. Johnson. *Pastoral Psychology* 1 (February 1950): 61-63.

_____. Review of *The Doctor and the Soul* by Victor E. Frankl. *Pastoral Psychology* 7 (June 1956): 65.

_____. Review of *Protestant Pastoral Counseling*, by O. H. Mowrer. *Christian Century*, 3 April 1963, pp. 430-31.

_____. "The Role of Religion in Psychoses." *Journal of Pastoral Care* 3 (Spring 1949): 21-30.

O'Brien, J. A. "Psychiatry and the Confessional." *Ecclesiastical Review* 98 (March 1938): 223-31.

Odenwald, Robert P. "Psychiatry and Psychoanalysis." *Sign* 29 (March 1950): 35-36.

_____. "Psychiatry and the Church: No Blanket Condemnation." *Catholic Charities Review* 40 (July 1946): 149-50.

Oraison, Marc. "Psychoanalysis and Confession." *Commonweal* 16 January 1959, pp. 424-25.

_____. "Psychoanalyst and the Confessor." *Cross Currents*, Fall 1958, pp. 63-76.

O'Reilly, Charles T., and O'Reilly, Edward J. "Religious Beliefs of Catholic College Students and Their Attitudes Towards Minorities." *Journal of Abnormal Psychology* 4 (1954): 378-80.

"Origins of Clinical Pastoral Training." *Pastoral Psychology* 4 (October 1953): 13-15.

Ostow, Mortimer. "The Nature of Religious Controls." *American Psychologist* 13 (1958): 71-74.

Outler, Albert. "Christian Context for Counseling." *Journal of Pastoral Care* 2 (Spring 1948): 1-12.

Overstreet, W. Bonaro. "The Unloving Personality and Religion of Love." *Pastoral Psychology* 4 (May 1953): 14-20.

Pacella, Bernard L. "A Critical Appraisal of Pastoral Counseling." *American Journal of Psychiatry* 123 no. 6 (1966): 646-51.

Paollome, Nathaniel. "Adjustment, Adaptation and the Sane Society." *Catholic Counselor* 8 (Fall 1963): 8-12.

Parker, Duane. "Pastoral Consultation Through a Community Mental Health Center." *Pastoral Psychology* 17 (May 1966): 42-47.

Parsons, Howard L. "Students at Six Colleges and Universities." *Religious Education* 58 no. 6 (1963): 538-44.

"Pastoral Psychology Retrospect." Editorial. *Pastoral Psychology* 4 (November 1953): 15.

Patrick, Sr. "Identifying the Emotionally Disturbed." *Catholic School Journal* 65 (October 1965): 47-48.

Pattison, A. Mansell. "Functions of the Clergy in the Community Mental Health Centers." *Pastoral Psychology* 16 (May 1965): 21-26.

Peters, M. Richard. "Study of the Intercorrelation of Personality Traits Among a Group of Novices in Religious Communities." *Catholic Educational Review* 47 (January 1949): 40.

Peterson, G. "Regression in Healing and Salvation." *Pastoral Psychology* 19 (September 1968): 33-39.

Peterson, N. C. and Farms, Beverly. "Group Dynamics Found in Scriptures." *Group Psychotherapy* 15 no. 2 (1962): 126-28.

Pfuetze, Paul E. "The Concept of Self in Contemporary Psychotherapy." *Pastoral Psychology* 9 (February 1958): 9-19.

Pinch, Stuart M. and Kroor, Edwin H. "Some Educational Factors in the Religious Education of Children." *Religious Education* 54 (1959): 36-43.

Pius XII, Pope. "Moral Limits of Medical Research and Treatment." Address to the First International Congress on the Histopathology of the Nervous System. 14 September 1952.

_____. "Morality and Applied Psychology." Address to the Congress of the International Association of Applied Psychology. Rome, 10 April 1958.

_____. "On Psychotherapy." Address to the Meeting of the International College of Neuro-Psychopharmacology. Rome, 9 September 1958.

Pixley, Emma and Beekman, Emma. "City Schools: The Faith of Youth as Shown by a Survey in Public Schools of Los Angeles." *Religious Education* 44 (1949): 336-42.

Polatin, Phillip. "Children and Divorce." *Pastoral Psychology* 9 (October 1958): 33-40.

"Pope Pius XII on Psychoanalysis." *America*, 89. 2 May 1953, p. 126.

Preston, Robert A. "A Chaplain Looks at Psychiatry." *Bulletin of the Menninger Clinic* 14 (1950): 22-26.

Pruyser, Paul W. "Psychological Examination: Augustine." *Journal for the Scientific Study of Religion* 5 (1965): 284-89.

Queener, E. Llewenllyn. "The Psychological Training of Ministers." *Pastoral Psychology* 7 (October 1956): 29-34.

Ramsey, Glenn V. "Aids for the Minister in Detecting Early Maladjustment." *Pastoral Psychology* 14 (February 1963): 41-51.

Review of *The Meaning of Religious Anxiety*, A Doctoral Dissertation by Fred Berthold. *Pastoral Psychology* 7 (February 1956): 50-52.

Rhodes, Lewis A. "Authoritarianism and Fundamentalism of Rural and Urban High School Students." *Journal of Educational Sociology* 34 (1960): 97-105.

Roberts, David E. "Cooperation Between Religion and Psychotherapy." *Pastoral Psychology* 1 (May 1950): 23-27.

_____. "Theological and Psychiatric Interpretations of Human Nature." *Journal of Pastoral Care* 1 (Winter 1947): 11-18.

_____. "When is Counseling or Psychotherapy Religious?" *Journal of Pastoral Care* 5 (Summer 1952): 1-18.

Rogers, Carl. "Divergent Trends in Methods of Improving Adjustment." *Pastoral Psychology* 1 (September 1950): 11-18.

Rogers, William F. "Needs of the Bereaved." *Pastoral Psychology* 1 (July 1950): 17-21.

_____. "The Pastor's Work with Grief." *Pastoral Psychology* 14 (September 1963): 19-26.

Róheim, G. "Animism and Religion," *Psychoanalytic Quarterly* 1 (1932): 59-112.

Rosenberg, Milton. "The Social Sources of the Current Religious Revival." *Pastoral Psychology* 8 (June 1957): 31-36.

Rosenthal, Hattie. "Psychotherapy for the Dying." *Pastoral Psychology* 14 (June 1963): 50-56.

Rosenzweig. E. M. "Minister and Congregation – A Study in Ambivalence." *Psychoanalytic Review* 28 (1941): 218-27.

Rumaud, J. "Psychologists vs. Morality." *Cross Currents* 1 (Winter 1951): 26-38.

Rutledge, Aaron L. "Concepts of God Among the Emotionally Upset." *Pastoral Psychology* 2 (May 1951): 22-25.

Sachs, Hans. "At the Gates of Heaven." *American Imago* 4 (1947): 15-32.

Salzman, Leon D. "A Critique of Wilhelm Reich's Psychoanalytic Theories." *Journal of Pastoral Care* 9 (Autumn 1955): 153-61.

_____. "Guilt, Responsibility and the Unconscious." *Pastoral Psychology* 15 (November 1964): 17-26.

_____. "Morality of Psychoanalysis." *Pastoral Psychology* 11 (March 1960): 24-29.

Savin, Aaron, "Self-Acceptance of Jewishness by Young Jewish People." *Jewish Education* 26 (December 1955): 22-31.

Scharfenberg, Joachim. "The Babylonian Captivity of Pastoral Theology." *Journal of Pastoral Care* 8 (Fall 1954): 125-34.

Scheeva, B. "Religion Marries Psychiatry." *Catholic World* 170 (December 1949): 161-65.

Schnitzer, Jeshaia, "Rabbis and Counseling." *Jewish Social Studies* 20 (1958): 131-52.

Schoelfield, H. R. "Psychoanalysis and the Parish Ministry." Address. *Journal of Religion and Health* 2 (January 1963): 112-28.

Schommer, John Kasa. "Participation, Religious Knowledge and Scholastic Aptitude." *Journal for the Scientific Study of Religion* 1 (1961): 88-97.

Selinger, Robert V. "Religious and Similar Experiences and Revelations in Patients with Alcohol Problems." *Journal of Clinical Psychotherapy* 7-8 (1947): 728-31.

Shaw, Don C. "Some General Considerations of the Religious Care of the Mentally Ill." *Journal of Clinical Pastoral Work* 1 no. 2 (1947): 20-25.

Sheenland, Roger. "The Development of a Religious Neuroticism Inventory." *Proceedings of the Christian Association for Psychological Studies* (April 1968): 96-106.

Sheldon, W. H. "Nature of the Human Mind and Body." *American Catholic Philosophical Association Proceedings* 13 (December 1937): 147-60.

Smith, M. C. and Barthurst, J. E. "Tests and Measurement in Religious Education." *Religious Education* 27 (1932): 439-42.

Smith, Philip M. "Prisoners' Attitudes Toward Organized Religion." *Religious Education* 51 (1956): 462-64.

Snow, John H. "Understanding 'Troublesome' Behavior in Children." *Journal of Pastoral Care* 13 (Spring 1959): 1-12.

Southard, Samuel. "The Evangelism of Children." *Pastoral Psychology* 7 (December 1956): 31-37.

Stafford, J. W. "Freedom in Experimental Psychology." *American Catholic Philosophical Association Proceedings* 16 (1940): 148-54.

_____. "Undergraduate Preparation for Clinical Psychology." Bibliography. *Catholic Educational Review* 47 (February 1949): 83-91.

Stander, A. "Science Behind Psychiatry." *Integrity* 4 (August 1950): 32-38.

Steck, M. "Thomistic Psychology and Freud's Psychoanalysis." *Thomist* 21 (April 1958): 25-45.

Steinhal, E. "Physician and the Minister." *Lutheran Quarterly* 2 (August 1950): 287-96.

Stendin, M. "Psychology Without a Soul," *Catholic World* 131 (July 1930): 131-44.

Stern, Karl. "Religion, Philosophy and Psychiatry." *Guild of Catholic Psychiatrists Bulletin* 1 no. 2 (December 1952): 18-23.

_____. "Religion and Psychiatry." *Commonweal*, 22 October 1948, pp. 30-33.

Stevic, P. R. "A Study in Feelings of Conformity in Religion." *Religious Education* 28 (1933): 364-67.

Stewart, Charles William. "Divorce Shatters One's World View and Makes One Question Life's Meaning." *Pastoral Psychology* 14 (April 1963): 10-16.

Stinnette, Charles. "Reflections and Transformations," in "Dialogues and Comments on an Article by Alden, 'Revelation and Psychotherapy.'" *I Continuum* 2 no. 2 (1964): 85, 110.

Stock, M. E. "Some Moral Issues in Psychoanalysis." *Thomist* 23 (April 1960): 143-88.

Stokes, Walter. Review of *Dogma and Compulsion* by Theodor Reik. *Pastoral Psychology* 4 (April 1953): 65-66.

Strickland, Francis L. "Pastoral Psychology – A Retrospect." *Pastoral Psychology* 4 (October 1953): 9-12.

Strunk, Orlo, and Reed, Kenneth E. "The Learning of Empathy" *Journal of Pastoral Care* 14 (Spring 1960): 44-48.

Sullivan, P. "Why Catholics Prefer Catholic Psychiatrists." *America*, 9 February 1963. pp. 199-201.

Summo, A. "The Counselor and Individual Psychological Testing." *Catholic Counselor* 5 (Fall 1960): 1-3.

Taubes, Jacob. "Religion and the Future of Psychoanalysis." *Psychoanalysis* 4 (1957): 136-42.

Terhune, William B. "Religion and Psychiatry." *Journal of Pastoral Care* 2 no. 2 (1948): 15-21.

Thomas, John Rea. "Evaluation of Clinical Pastoral Training and 'Part Time' Training in General Hospital." *Journal of Pastoral Care* 12 (Spring 1957): 28-34.

Thompson, Clara. "Towards a Psychology of Women." *Pastoral Psychology* 4 (May 1953): 29-38.

Thorner, Isidor. "Ascetic Protestantism and Alcoholism." *Psychiatry* 16 (1953): 167-76.

Thouless, R. H. "Scientific Method in the Study of Psychology of Religion." *Character and Personality* 7 (1938): 103-8.

Tiebout, Harry M. "The Act of Surrender in the Treatment of the Alcoholic." *Pastoral Psychology* 1 (May 1950): 42-50.

_____. "Alcoholics Anonymous: An Experiment of Nature." *Pastoral Psychology* 13 (April 1962): 45-62.

Tillich, Paul. "The Impact of Pastoral Psychology on Theological Thought." *Pastoral Psychology* 11 (February 1960): 17-23.

_____. "Psychoanalysis, Existentialism and Theology." *Pastoral Psychology* 9 (October 1958): 9-17.

_____. Review of *Psychoanalysis and Religion* by Erich Fromm. *Pastoral Psychology* 2 (June 1951): 62.

Trueblood, David Elton. "The Challenge of Freud." *Pastoral Psychology* 9 (June 1958): 37-44.

VanderVeldt, James. "Religion and Mental Health." *Mental Hygiene* 35 (1951): 177-89.

Vaughn, Richard P. "Counseling the Former Nun." *National Catholic Guidance Counselors Journal* 9 (Winter 1965): 93-101.

_____. "The Neurotic Religious." *Review of Religious* 17 (1958): 271-78.

_____. "A Psychological Assessment Program for Candidates to the Religious Life." *American Catholic Psychological Association* 1 (February 1963): 65-70.

_____. "Refering Students to Psychiatrists and Psychologists." *Catholic Counselor* 3 (Winter 1959): 30-38.

Bibliography

Verdery, E. A. "Pastoral Care of the Alcoholic's Family After Sobriety." *Pastoral Psychology* 13 (April 1962): 30-38.

Walters, Orville S. "The Minister and the New Counseling." *Journal of Pastoral Care* 7 (Winter 1953): 191-203.

_____. "Psychiatrist and the Christian Faith." *Christian Century*, 20 July 1960, pp. 47-49.

_____. "Psychiatry-Religion Dialogue." *Christian Century*, 27 December 1961, pp. 155-59.

Warwick, C. A. "On Casting out a Devil." *America*, 15 November 1947, pp. 81-82.

Warwick, Le Roy A. "The Clergy as Marriage Counselors." *Journal of Religion and Health* 5 no. 3 (1966): 2-9.

Weger, George H., and Gerkin, Charles V. "A Religious Story Test: Some Findings with Delinquent Boys." *Journal of Pastoral Care* 7 no. 2 (1953): 77-90.

Wiegel, Gustave. "The Challenge of Peace" *Pastoral Psychology* 10 (February 1959) 29-36.

Weigert, Edith. "Love and Fear: A Psychological Interpretation." *Journal of Pastoral Care* 5 (Summer 1951): 12-22.

_____. "Psychiatry and Sin." *Journal of Pastoral Care* 4 no. 1-2 (1950): 43-49.

Weinstein, Jacob J. "Religion Looks at Psychiatry." *Pastoral Psychology* 9 (November 1958): 25-32.

Weir, E. W. "Summary of a Discussion of Scholastic Psychology and Modern Experimental Psychology." *American Catholic Philosophical Association Proceedings* 12 (December 1936): 109-11.

"What Can the Minister Reasonably Expect from a Psychiatrist or a Psychologist in Terms of the Latter's Dealing with Moral Principles in the Life of his Patient?" *Pastoral Psychology* 1 (March 1950): 55-56.

Whitcomb, John C. "The Relationship of Personality Characteristics of Ministers to Adjustment." *Religious Education* 52 (1957): 371-74.

White, Abridge V. "Can Psychologists be Religious?" *Commonweal*, 18 September 1953, pp. 583-84.

_____. "Place of Religion in Psychotherapy." *Catholic World* 162 (October 1945): 80-81.

Whitlock, Glenn E. "Choice of the Ministry as an Active or Passive Decision." *Pastoral Psychology* 12 (March 1961): 31-45.

_____. "Role and Self-Concepts in the Choice of the Ministry as a Vocation." *Journal of Pastoral Care* 17 (Winter 1963): 208-17.

Wieman, H. N. "How Religion Cures Human Ills." *Journal of Religion* 7 (May 1927): 263-76.

Wilkens, Walter. "Another Viewpoint on the Psychology of Personality Development." *Hospital Progress* 31 (October 1950): 314-16.

Williams, M. O. "The Psychological-Psychiatric Appraisal of Candidates for Missionary Service." *Pastoral Psychology* 9 (December 1958): 41-44.

Williams, Robert L., and Spurgion, Cole. "Religiosity, Generalized Anxiety and Apprehension Concerning Death." *Journal of Social Psychology* 75 no. 1 (1968): 11-17.

Williamson, C. H. "Danger of Psychoanalysis" *Catholic World* 136 (December 1932): 296-301.

Winter, Gibson, "Pastoral Counseling or Pastoral Care." *Pastoral Psychology* 8 (February 1957): 16-22.

Wise, Carroll A. "The Call to the Ministry." *Pastoral Psychology* 9 (December 1958):9-17

_____. "Education of the Pastor for Marriage Counseling." *Pastoral Psychology* 10 (December 1959):15-18

Woodruff, A. D. "Students' Verbalized Values." *Religious Education* 38 (1943): 321-24.

Woodward, Luther E. "Contributions of the Minister to Mental Hygiene." *Pastoral Psychology* 3 (February 1950): 19, (May 1950): 43-47.

Zellner, A. A. "Screening of Candidates for the Priesthood and Religious Life." *Catholic Educational Review* 58 (February 1960): 96-105.

Zilboorg, Gregory, "The Psychiatrist and the Problem of Religion." *Issues* 2 no. 2 (December 1954): 5-7.

_____. "Psychiatry's Moral Sphere." *America*, 3 June 1958. pp. 308-9.

Index

absence of religion as a cause of, 22
in Adlerian psychology, 18, 19
anxiety and, 87, 88, 89, 90, 91, 92, 93
attempts to measure, 151
in Catholic psychological theory, 62,
    64, 65, 67, 68, 82, 83, 99, 113, 159
the conversion experience and, 107
environment in curing, 31
in Fairbairn's psychological theory, 25
in Fromm's psychological theory, 29-
    30
grief and, 100, 101
in group therapy, 140, 141
guilt in, 93-94, 95-96, 97, 98, 99, 100,
    114, 158
in homosexuality, 135
in Horney's psychological theory, 28,
    44, 48, 54
in Jewish psychological theory, 75, 92,
    100
in Jungian psychology, 22, 58
love and, 103
masturbation and, 113
in May's psychological theory, 51, 52,
    87, 88
ministers and priests and, 142, 143,
    153
in Morris's psychological theory, 55
neo-Freudians and, 15, 53
in Protestant pastoral psychology, 39,
    40, 42, 46, 49
in Rankian psychology, 23
in Reich's psychological theory, 27
in Reik's psychological theory, 59
religion as seen by the early social
    scientists, 33
    by Freud, 13, 45, 46
    by Fromm, 30-31
sexual behavior and, 111
sin and, 98, 99, 100
in Sullivan's psychological theory, 48
theologians on, 78, 80, 81, 82, 83
Nichols, Roger B., on anxiety, 87
Niebuhr, Reinhold, 51
    on anxiety, 88, 90
    praise of Horney by, 54
Non-directive counseling, 138, 159
    group therapy as, 140
Nordberg, R.B., on rationality, 83
Noveck, Simon, 126
    argument for Jewish acceptance of
        Freudian psychology by, 74
    on grief, 102
Novis, K., on treatment of mental illness, 82
Nuns
    counseling for, 83
    psychological problems of, 143

psychological testing of, 148
Nursing schools, Catholic, psychological
    courses in, 146

Oates, Wayne E., 38, 43-44, 46-47, 160
    on anxiety, 89-90
    on ministerial counseling, 128, 138
    on prevention of mental illness, 124-25
Obedience
    in conversion experiences, 109
    doctrine of in Catholicism, 103
    theologians on, 78
Object-choice; object-cathexis, 10
Object relations. *See* Interpersonal relations
Object splitting
    in Fairbairn's psychological theory, 25
    in Klein's psychological theory, 23, 25
Occupations. *See* Employment
Odenwald, Robert P.
    on anxiety, 91
    argument for Catholic acceptance of
        Freudian psychology by, 62, 63,
        65-67
    on directive counseling, 138
    on guilt, 95-96
    on love, 103
    on priests as counselors, 129-30
    on psychosomatic illness, 144
    on sex education, 113
    on sin, 99
Oedipus complex, 11-12, 13, 110, 111,
    154
    the *Bar Mitzvah* and, 33
    conversion and, 108
    in Freud's (Anna) psychological theory,
        24
    in Fromm's psychological theory, 30
    Hiltner on, 42
    in Jewish psychological theory, 73, 74
    in Jungian psychology, 21
    in Klein's psychological theory, 23
    among primitive people, 33
    in Rankian psychology, 22
    in Reich's psychological theory, 27
Oliver, J.R., on sexual behavior, 110
Optimism, of Individual Psychology, 17
Oraison, Marc, argument for Catholic
    acceptance of Freudian psychology
    by, 68
Oral stage (in personality development), 11
    Fromm's receptive character related to,
        30
    neo-Freudians and, 15
    teaching about in religious education,
        146
Orgasm, in Reich's psychological theory, 59
Original sin. *See* Sin

Religion
  absence of in creating psychoses, 22
  in allaying alienation and anxiety, 29,
    31, 60
  Freudian and neo-Freudian psychology
    in, 7-15, 85-87, 114-15, 117-49
    anxiety and, 87-93
    Catholic Church and, 61-71, 81-84,
      91, 95-96, 98-99, 101, 103, 104,
      105, 106, 108, 113-14, 115, 144,
      152-53, 156-57, 159
    conversion and, 106-9
    early social scientists' studies of, 33-
      35
    forgiveness and, 104
    grief and, 100-102
    guilt and, 93-97
    Judaism and, 71-77, 84, 91-93, 96-
      97, 99-100, 101, 103-4, 105,
      106, 109, 153, 156, 157, 159
    love and, 102-4
    mysticism and, 105-6
    from 1965-1978, 151-62
    in the Progressive era, 1-5, 153
    salvation and, 104-105
    sexual behavior and, 109-14
    sin and, 97-100
    theologians on, 77-84
  James's theory of, 2-4
    in Jungian psychology, 22, 56, 57,
      58-59
    primitive seen in psychoanalytic
      terms, 13, 33
    reduction of to measurable percep-
      tions, 2
    regressive nature of, 35
    Thouless on the psychology of, 5
  See also Fundamentalism; Pastoral
    psychology, Protestant; Pente-
    costal sects; Protestantism; names
    of denominations (e.g., Episcopal
    Church)
Religion and science, 154-55. *See also*
  Social scientists
Religious education, 144-49, 161
Religious Education, 38
Repentance. *See* Penance and repentance
Repression
  in anxiety states, 88, 90
  as a defense mechanism, 10
  in May's psychological theory, 52
  the Oedipus complex and, 11
  in Reich's psychological theory, 27
  religious education as, 144, 145
  of the sex instinct, 112, 151
Resistance and transference, 12, 98, 152
  in Catholic psychological theory, 83

  in Freud's (Anna) psychological theory,
    25
  in group therapy, 140, 141
  in Jungian psychology, 22
  in Klein's psychological theory, 23
Responsibility
  in Catholic psychological theory, 66
  in Fromm's psychological theory, 56
  in group therapy, 140
  inability of the neurotic to assume, 44
  in May's psychological theory, 51
Retarded, ministerial counseling for, 136
Review of Religion, 39
Ritual
  Catholic, 152
  in Jewish psychological theory, 75
    guilt and, 97
  in primitive man, 13
  See also Ceremony
Roberts, David E., 39-40, 79, 160
  *Psychotherapy and a Christian View of
    Man* by, 41
Rogers, Carl, 50, 128
  Brevis's use of, 139
  criticism of by Bioren, 138
  on grief, 100, 101
  influence on Stinnette, 53
  praise of by Walters, 79
  psychological theories of, 51
Róheim, G., 33
Roman Catholic Church
  as a creator of fears and repression, 44
  Freudian psychology and, 61-71, 81-
    84, 152-53, 156-57, 159
    anxiety, 91
    conversion, 108
    grief, 101
    guilt, 95-96
    love, 103, 104, 115
    mysticism, 105
    psychosomatic illness, 144
    sexual behavior, 113-14
    sin, 98-99
    worship service, 106
  Jung on, 59
  religious education in, 146
  testing programs, 148-49
  See also Nuns; Priests
Rorschach test, 147
Rosenberg, Milton, 80
Rosenzweig, E.M., 34
Rumaud, J., argument for Catholic accep-
  tance of Freudian psychology by, 63
Rural areas, need for therapeutic help in,
  161
Rutledge, Aaron L., on ministering to
  people with personality problems, 135

psychology, 61, 67, 69
Thompson, Clara
  on the changing status of women, 59
  influence of Rank on, 23
Thorner, Isidor, on anxiety, 89
Thought and thinking, in Jungian psychology, 21
Thouless, R.H., psychology of religion of, 5
Tiebout, Harry M., on conversion, 107, 108
Tillich, Paul, 38, 155
  on Fromm, 55
  psychological theories of, 51-52, 55-56
    anxiety in, 88, 90
Totemic religion, ritualistic killing in, 13
Totalitarianism
  attraction to by May's dependent individual, 52
  influence on Jewish psychological theory, 73-74
  submission eventually leading to, 27
  See also Dictatorships
Trances, James's ideas on in religious conversion, 4
Trueblood, David Elton, 80
Truth
  in Fromm's psychological theory, 55, 56
  Hiltner on, 42
  in Jungian psychology, 22

Unconscious
  in Boisen's psychological theory, 57
  bringing of to the conscious mind, 42
  in Catholic psychological theory, 62, 63, 64, 65, 66, 67, 69, 81, 82, 83, 152
  in existential psychology, 50
    May's, 50, 52
    Tillich's, 51
  guilt in the, 93, 94, 95
  as the home for wishes, 9
  in Jewish psychological theory, 73, 74
  in Jungian psychology, 20, 21, 58
  in May's psychological theory, 53
  in Protestant pastoral psychology, 45, 48
  sexual behavior and, 152
  sin and, 98
  in Sullivan's psychological theory, 26
  See also Subconscious
Union of American Hebrew Congregations, 149
U.S. Federal Bureau of Prisons, chaplaincy program in (1930s), 120
U.S. National Institute of Health, 131
U.S. Works Progress Administration, 146

Values and attitudes
  in Adlerian psychology, 18
  in Catholic psychological theory, 68
  in existential psychology, 50
    May's, 51
  in group therapy, 140, 141
  guilt and, 96
  inner in Jungian psychology, 21
  in Jewish psychological theory, 72, 96
  sexual, 111
  in Sullivan's psychological theory, 26
  testing for in Judaism, 149
    in Protestantism, 148
  See also Morality and ethics
Vandervelt, James
  on anxiety, 91
  argument for Catholic acceptance of Freudian psychology by, 63, 65-67
  on directive counseling, 138
  on guilt, 95-96
  on love, 103
  on priests as counselors, 129-30
  on psychosomatic illness, 144
  on sex education, 113
  on sin, 99
Verdery, E.A., on ministering to alcoholics, 134
Veterans hospitals
  chaplains in, 133
  clinical training programs in, 121-22
Victorian period
  guilt in, 94
  influence on Freud, 57
  sexual morality in, 52, 110
  women in, 59
Vienna Psychoanalytic Society, 22

Walters, Orville S., 80-81
  on Rogerian therapy, 79
War, threat of as a creator of anxiety, 90. *See also* World War I; World War II
Warwick, Le Roy A., on priests as marriage counselors, 152-53
Weber, Carlo, on psychological problems of priests and nuns, 152
Weigel, Gustave, on the conflict between psychiatrists and theologians, 68
Weigert, Edith H.
  on love, 103
  on sin, 98
Weinstein, Jacob J., 75
Weir, E.W., argument for Catholic acceptance of Freudian psychology by, 61
White, Abridge V., argument for Catholic acceptance of Freudian psychology by, 62, 63
Weiman, H.N., on salvation, 77

Wilberforce, William, social adjustment of, 79
Will
  in existential psychology, 50
  surrender of in religious conversion, 3
Williams, M.O., on psychological testing of ministers, 143
Williams, Robert L., 151
Williamson, C.H., 81
Willoughby, R.R., on anxiety, 87
Winchester, B.S., on religious education, 145
Winter, Gibson, 80
Wise, Carroll A., 47
  on ministerial therapy, 127
  on psychological testing of ministers, 143
  on sexual behavior, 113
Wishes
  religion in fulfilling, 13
  unconscious as the home of, 9
Withdrawal, in Horney's psychological theory, 28. *See also* Regression
Women
  effect of employment on morality of, 86
  sexuality of, 110, 112
  Thompson on changing roles of, 59
Woodward, Luther E., 38
Worcester State Hospital, 119

Word association test, 22
World War I, influence of Freud's theories, 8, 9
World War II
  in creating new interest in Freudian psychology, 37, 39, 41, 42, 85-86, 87, 154-55
  among Catholics, 62
  among Jews, 73-74
  effect on children, 136
  neurotic reactions in the era following, 52
  psychological testing in, 147
Worship
  as a counseling technique, 138
  in curing psychosomatic illness, 144
  effect of Freud on religious conceptions of, 86
  function of in mental hospitals, 133
  psychological theories on useful to theology, 106

Yellowless, D., on St. Paul, 110
Yeshiva University, 130-31

Zilboorg, Gregory, argument for Catholic acceptance of Freudian psychology by, 64, 67, 70